Recovery from CFS

50 Personal Stories

Compiled and edited

by

Alexandra Barton

authorHOUSE®

AuthorHouse™ UK Ltd.
500 Avebury Boulevard
Central Milton Keynes, MK9 2BE
www.authorhouse.co.uk
Phone: 08001974150

First published by AuthorHouse   4/28/2008

ISBN: 978-1-4343-6358-9 (sc)

Printed in the United States of America
Bloomington, Indiana

This book is printed on acid-free paper.

Cover photograph of Anna Hemmings winning a World Championship Gold Medal nine months after recovering from CFS (see Anna's story).

Image by Mark Watson: www.inciteimages.com

This book is dedicated to everyone with CFS/ME and their carers

20% book proceeds to CFS/ME research

Thank You

To all the contributors who have given their time and energy writing their stories of hope for this book.

To my husband and two children, who were always there for me and who gave me the best reason in the world to get well. To my parents, for providing me with a comforting, twenty-four hour telephone support line and many words of wisdom.

To my friend Clare, whose story is in the book, for buoying up my hope when I needed it.

Note to reader

This book should not be used as an alternative to appropriate medical care and before following any self-help advice given in this book readers are urged to consult a qualified medical specialist. There are no proven treatments for CFS/ME and no guarantee that any of the treatments and therapies mentioned in this book will work for anybody other than the author. The authors are not advocating any 'cures', they are simply describing what, if any, therapies helped them most on their own personal journeys to recovery. The authors and publishers cannot accept legal responsibility for any problem arising out of experimentation with any of the methods or therapies described.

CFS and ME are generally thought of as the same illness but are referred to using the different terms by different authors.

CONTENTS

Foreword

A fifty-first success story - how you CAN get well now!

As Alexandra Barton lovingly proves in this excellent book, people with chronic fatigue syndrome, myalgic encephalomyelitis and fibromyalgia *can clearly recover* and do best when both the physical and psycho-spiritual issues are treated simultaneously. In this excellent book, fifty CFS patients offer hope and insights from their own personal journeys, so that people can begin on their own road to recovery. This is critical, as there is so much ignorance, misinformation, and downright hostility in the standard medical community when it comes to these syndromes.

I am happy to be the 'fifty-first success story'. I know what you've been through. 1975 was a really rough year. I was caught in the middle of a family melt down while in my third year of medical school. I was twenty-two and my father had died years earlier, so I was paying my own way. Finally the stress caught up with me. I had what I called the 'drop dead flu'. Three months later I was still exhausted, unable to sleep, achy all over and had no brain. Devastated, I had to drop out of medical school. As I was paying my own way and relying on scholarships, student loans and work, which I was now too sick to do, I found myself homeless and sleeping in parks. This was to be my introduction to chronic fatigue syndrome and fibromyalgia.

By working on both my physical and psychological issues, I achieved a full recovery. The illness actually became a blessing which taught me to get touch with my own feelings and desires. I live a very busy life now making effective treatment available for everyone - and moving at optimal speed is a lot healthier if you are going in the right direction!

So what is causing CFS/FMS/ME? I do not view these syndromes as the enemy. Rather, I see them as attempts on the body's part to protect itself from further harm and damage, in the face of any of a number of overwhelming stresses. A simple way to look at CFS/FMS/ME would be to view them like a circuit breaker in a house. When certain systems are over-stressed, the circuit breaker will go off to prevent damage to the home's wiring.

In milder cases, your 'circuit breaker' can come back on and systems can return to healthy function simply by supplying the body with rest and proper nutrition. In CFS/FMS/ME, however, it is as if the main circuit breaker (in this situation the hypothalamus- a master gland in the brain) has malfunctioned. When this occurs, rest is no longer enough to restore proper function.

Despite the many diverse triggers that can cause these syndromes, most patients' symptoms seem to come from a common end-point - excessive energy demands resulting in dysfunction of the hypothalamic 'circuit breaker'. This area controls sleep, hormonal function, temperature regulation and the autonomic nervous system (e.g. blood pressure, blood flow, sweating, and movement of food through the bowel). The hypothalamic dysfunction by itself can therefore cause most of the symptoms we see in these patients.

So both physical and situational stresses can cause me to 'blow a fuse'? Absolutely! As is the case with other illnesses, for example heart attacks, the trigger can be physical and/or psychological stresses. In fact, anything that results in you overdrawing your 'energy account' can trigger the process. Once you've blown the fuse, you're most likely to get well when you treat both the physical and psychological 'energy drainers'. A number of books expertly address how to treat the physical component of these syndromes and some also address the psycho-spiritual steps you can take to reclaim your health - an area you have full power over. Reporting on how both approaches can help is one of the strengths of "Recovery from CFS - 50 Personal Stories".

Joseph Campbell summarized the road to health well when he said "Follow Your Bliss!" By paying close attention to what makes you *feel good* and choosing to focus on and do only these things, whilst also getting the medical treatment you need, you will dramatically speed your recovery.

The good news is that fibromyalgia, chronic fatigue syndrome and myalgic encephalomyelitis are now *very* treatable, although most physicians are not yet familiar with the newest research on effective treatment and it is best to see a doctor who specializes in CFS/FMS/ME. To improve and even get well - and research shows that over 85% of you can - it is important that you start by realizing the importance of treating these syndromes' *underlying causes,* and not only the symptoms. In fact, our landmark placebo controlled study showed an average 91% improvement by simply treating sleep, hormonal support, infections, and giving optimized nutritional support. The full study can be seen at www.vitality101.com.

Getting from where you are now to where you want to be is easier with the right guidance, however. Alexandra Barton has taken on the important task of showing you how you can recover by treating both the physical and psycho-spiritual components of these illnesses, whilst offering you resources for you to explore. As you read this book, make notes of those things that *feel* best to you, and begin with those. Prepare to be empowered!

Wishing you all of God's blessings and love and best wishes for a full recovery.

Jacob Teitelbaum MD
Medical director of the National Fibromyalgia and Fatigue Centers, USA

Introduction

I had CFS/ME for twelve years and it devastated my home life, my social life and my career. For five years I was housebound and on the rare occasion I did go out I needed a wheelchair or disabled scooter. We had a full-time, live-in au-pair to help look after the children and the house and, needless to say, I got very depressed. What I wanted most in life was to create a happy family and to be a good mum, but instead I was an invalid and a burden on my husband and children.

I also got depressed because I couldn't find people who had recovered. Everywhere I looked I found people who had had CFS for many, many years. I rang support lines only to be told that the best I could hope for was to be able to 'manage' my illness. I went to local support groups, to find them full of people who had been ill for at least ten years. And there was, and still is, a popular view that CFS is 'incurable' – which didn't help at all. What I really needed to know was that it was *possible* to recover from CFS/ME. I needed to hear about people who had recovered and how they had done it. I needed to believe that I could recover, because, without hope there is only despair, and how can you carry on with only despair for company? I had to know that there was hope of a future worth living in order to keep going!

When I couldn't find that hope I had to manufacture it for myself. I looked for inspirational recovery stories from other illnesses and I tried anything and everything that I thought might help me to get better. Everything I tried gave me the hope that I needed to keep going. And I did eventually recover. I was once again able to lead a normal life, to be a wife and mother and keep house and return to work. I was able to go on active family holidays, camping and canoeing in the Ardeche in France, sailing in Greece and cycling thirteen miles in a day in Cornwall.

I realised then that what I wanted to do was bring the hope that I had so desperately needed when I was ill to all those people who were still suffering from CFS/ME. I decided that the best way to do this would be to find other people who had recovered and ask them if they would write their stories. I wanted to let everybody know that recovery *is* possible, how we had done it and that if we could do it so could they. I began to look for other people who had returned to a normal life. I advertised in local newspapers and magazines in the UK and abroad, and in my search for stories I realised that CFS/ME is only considered 'incurable' because the medical profession don't have a 'cure' for it. It doesn't mean that it is impossible to get well! People do get better and the reason we don't hear about them is because the vast majority disappear back into normal life, no longer maintaining links with the world of CFS/ME.

I found many people who had recovered, and fifty of them agreed to write their stories. The result is this book. If you have CFS/ME or care for someone with CFS/ME, this book is written for you. I hope that this simple collection of stories will help you to see that not only is a full recovery possible, but that reading about other people's return to a normal life will at the very least cheer you up when you are feeling down and give you a lift when you need it.

The contributors to this book and I wish you all the very, very best for your own recovery.

Alexandra Barton

The Elephant and M.E.

What it is like to have CFS/ME

Imagine feeling dreadful with the flu – really-off work dreadful, having-to-be in-bed dreadful. You feel *horrible*. Your muscles ache and are all weak and wobbly. You know the feeling, it's like walking on two sticks of jelly when you've just completed a marathon. You feel completely drained – not just tired and exhausted but utterly drained. Your head feels spaced out, dizzy, filled with a thick black fog and you just can't think. Noise drives you mad. You feel SO ill that you wish you were dead. And then, imagine that on top of all that, you have to carry on your back the biggest elephant you have ever seen, and that the elephant is there to stay for a very, very, very long time.

He will accompany you to bed. He will accompany you to the bathroom. In fact, he will accompany you wherever you go from now on. Everything you do, which seems so simple to everybody else, feels to you as if you are climbing Mount Everest with a ten ton elephant on your back - whilst suffering from flu – even if you are just walking a few yards. Even if you are just sitting down. Why else do people with ME need a rest every few minutes? You would too if you were that sick and were carrying an elephant. Why do people with ME cry? You would too!

That's what living with ME is like. The only thing that changes along the way is that at various stages the elephant gets either heavier or lighter. Towards your recovery, the elephant sometimes hops off for a short while, but you can guarantee that after you've let loose with whoops of joy as the elephant goes off elsewhere, he soon returns, bigger and heavier than he was before because he's replenished himself with a big dinner, and you've worn yourself out with the excitement, so he now weighs far more than he did. And until you've been travelling up that mountain a few more days or weeks or months, practising rigid pacing discipline and not allowing yourself to get upset or stressed (heaven forbid) at the weight you are carrying, he continues to weigh at least a ton or more.

Then the day comes (if you're not feeding him) that he gets lighter, then hungry, and off he jumps. You, released suddenly from your prison, again go completely berserk with joy, forgetting entirely that the elephant has only just gone around the corner for dinner and that he even exists at all. But he is coming back. Oh yes, he's coming back. And again, he returns bigger and heavier than he was before.

Sometimes he comes back lighter. But that all depends on you. If you don't go wild with joy when he jumps off, if you restrain yourself and continue to live as if he *was* on your back even though he isn't (and who wants to do that?) then he might come back lighter than before.

Over time. Time, time, time. The poor person with ME – how can you be comforted with getting better over 'time'? How much time? The rest of your life? But yes, over time, the person with ME begins to get stronger (if of course, they're remembering to do the one hundred and one things they're supposed to do right – eat right, exercise right, be happy (!) have regular rests and so on) and then the elephant gets lighter and hops off more often. And then one day the elephant hops off one more time and doesn't bother to return. And isn't that just wonderful?! Freedom, happiness and health are yours again. Beware though - if you haven't been a good boy or girl and (like me) you didn't learned the lessons you should have learned in elephant school – then one day, when you least expect it, he will come charging around the corner in a fury – and he will jump on you – and you will be flattened – and then you and he will be a team again. And, however much

2

you cry and wail it will do no good at all, because the elephant is determined that until you know *why* he is with you, he will stay with you again, and keep coming back, until you do.

Alexandra Barton

Margaret's Story

The wheelchair, the stick and the tin of Jersey Royals

In 1985 I left college and worked as a beauty therapist for six years. In 1991 at twenty-eight, I started my own salon. I had a happy, busy year running on what I now recognise was adrenaline. I was (and still am) a do-er. For example, when I had an hour or two to spare in the salon I popped over to my grandmother's house and redecorated her bathroom. I considered myself fit and had no viral or bacterial infections, yet, over the course of that year, I wound down like a clockwork toy. One evening, I got home, slid down the wall to the floor and didn't get up for two weeks. My mind wanted to get up but my body didn't. My body won.

I was fortunate to be diagnosed with ME straight away by my General Practitioner. This was because a doctor in the practice was a sufferer. He gave me the number of a national support group and advised rest. In 1991 I knew nothing about ME except that yachtswoman Clare Francis suffered from it and I vaguely remembered her mentioning something about depression in an interview. I felt confused. I wasn't depressed, my body had stopped working. No one could believe that I had given up work just like that, but the truth was that it had given me up. The support group was helpful but no one seemed to know what ME was or how I was supposed to get rid of it. In the end I took my GP's advice - I rested and awaited recovery.

I spent my days on a sun-lounger in my living-room thinking, in a bit, when I feel better, I'll get up. I couldn't sit on a dining chair. I was too tired to sleep. Three years later I was still there feeling just as exhausted. Time didn't drag; I wasn't bored, I was exhausted. It took me several days to work up the energy to water a wilting houseplant. I would stare at it day after day thinking, tomorrow, I'll manage to water it tomorrow.

Niceties such as bathing ceased. I couldn't hold up a telephone receiver, eat soup or stand up for the time it took a tea bag to brew. Andy, my husband, took over the cooking - but not the dusting, men can't see dust. I got a home help. Clothes consisted of a tracksuit in the cold and a cheesecloth dress in the warm. Remember that there is no law to say you must wear underwear.

I soon solved the hygiene problem. I got into Andy's evening bath. More often than not he was still in it, but it's very difficult to prevent somebody stepping into your bath and besides - it gave us a nice opportunity for me to chat about all the things I hadn't been able to do that day. Thankfully, Andy took my illness in his stride and it strengthened our relationship rather than damaged it.

Every muscle felt sore even though I hadn't gone anywhere. I began using a stick - mostly because it stopped self-important types of various sexes and ages, from bumping into what appeared to be a twenty-eight year-old woman. If you don't like the look of a stick, a walking stick umbrella is the answer. However, if you rely on it too much and it rains, prepare to get wet.

I took to sitting down in queues. Nobody paid much attention - with the exception of one elderly gentleman who enquired whether I wished to know the direction of Mecca.

During this time, I embarked on my own form of energy conservation. I invested in an electric food processor, tin opener, blender, juicer, carrot grater, toothbrush and fly swatter. If it had a plug on it, I bought it. I also bought an orange peeler, apple corer, toothpaste squeezer, pill-crusher and letter-opener (non-electric sadly). I even got my houseplants rigged up to an automatic irrigation system.

I put the iron in the loft (where it still resides) and bought Lycra clothes and seersucker table and bed linen and moved to a bungalow. If you can't get out, send off for it. Nowadays, practically everything you need can be bought on Ebay. Fund your Ebay purchases by selling all that stuff in the back of the cupboard you thought you needed but didn't.

As well as fatigue, I had severe hypoglycaemia, which meant I could only go a certain length of time between meals. When I did leave the house, I always took a snack with me and since I was trying to balance my sugar intake to avoid my blood sugar yo-yoing, this took the form of a can of Jersey new potatoes and a tin opener. However, I don't recommend this as it does tend to ruin the shape of your handbag.

I also suffered from gut problems ranging from an upset stomach from eating half an orange to the inability to digest anything except poached chicken and boiled potatoes.

I wouldn't say I got depressed. Frustrated, I did get. Every time I saw a large expanse of glass, I had the urge to hurl something through it. Memory loss was also a problem. Now what was I saying? Oh yes… my mind would blank mid-thought and I had to use phrases such as 'window obscuring material' for curtain. There were advantages to having no short-term memory. I would often happen upon a lovely cup of tea that someone had thoughtfully made me. It wasn't too difficult to work out who the kind and thoughtful person turned out to be, since I was alone in the house.

I found reading or watching television exhausting and filled my time listening to talking books or writing. I went out once a week in a wheelchair with a head and footrest. However, being pushed around by a selection of relatives is extremely frustrating, however lovely the relatives. I have every sympathy for pushchair-bound children who scream to be let out.

Things got better when I discovered Shop Mobility. They will lend you an electric wheelchair or scooter for free and, since a wheelchair trumps a pushchair, you get to mow through all those brain-dead mums who select the middle of the pavement as a good spot in which to have a natter. That's worth it just in itself. Do be careful though as you're freewheeling through clothing aisles. I once accidentally shoplifted a purple and silver thong that attached itself to the handle of my wheelchair. I returned it of course – much to Andy's regret. I also once shoplifted a pin cushion, it fell down the arm of my coat and wedged there as I was reaching for something on a high self. I only discovered it when I got home. But enough of my career as an accidental shoplifter.

Being in a wheelchair does tend to bring out the overly helpful side of people's natures. On a family outing, we happened upon a teddy bear museum that everyone fancied visiting. Everyone except me. In my opinion, stuffed toys are a waste of fluff. I was quite relieved when the museum turned out to be inaccessible to wheelchairs. The lady at the reception desk was excessively apologetic, my parents were suitably indignant. The receptionist offered to fetch a few out for me to look at. It was a tough job convincing everyone that I really didn't want to look at any bears.

During this time, I prided myself on trying absolutely no alternative therapies whatsoever. If I had spare money, which I didn't, I spent it on carrot juice.

Three years down the line I happened, by chance, to hear of Dr. David Smith. Apparently, he had an effective treatment for ME that wasn't going on fair rides or snapping yourself out of it. I got a doctor's referral and treatment began on the NHS.

It was horribly simple - SSRI's (also used as antidepressants) to 'alter my brain chemistry' and a graded activity programme. Notice I say 'activity' not 'exercise'. In my case, activity consisted of walking to the end of my drive and back everyday. Needless to say, I had tried 'activity' but I'd gone too far, too fast, too soon, for too long. The key to success was the *graded* bit. At no time did I push myself to exhaustion. Dr. Smith told me that recovery wasn't going to be easy, but it was, actually. You stick to the programme: you get better. Over the course of around twelve months, I got sufficiently better to live some kind of life again. The most difficult part was having the patience to wait.

My recovery was a steady climb. Having said that, I had an excellent carer in my husband and no external pressures such as children or work to cope with. I don't know if the medication helped but it didn't hinder, had no nasty side effects, and was no problem to stop. Dr. Smith gets one hell of a nice Christmas card every year.

For a few years, I felt at a loss as to how to describe myself. I was an independent businesswoman turned invalid. Not nice. While you are recovering I recommend turning a hobby into your new 'profession'. In other words, make something and sell a few. When you find yourself well enough to attend a social function someone will ask the inevitable question: "And what do you do?" You can then answer: "I am a greetings card maker/jewellery designer/writer/painter." They need not know that you only managed to shift one handmade greetings card to Aunty Mavis for a total of 25p. (Aunty Mavis drives a hard bargain). If someone pays you for your skills - that makes you a professional.

In the last stages of recovery I became slightly mentally unhinged. This took the form of severe anxiety. While I was physically disabled I just existed. Once I began to get better the world came back for me to deal with. I distinctly remember not being able to drive to the corner shop to buy a bottle of milk.

My state of mind was largely rectified by a counsellor at my GP's surgery, who pointed out that rather than me being a feeble, pathetic jelly-woman, I was, in fact, a bit of a hero and coping rather well - everything considered. I have continued to think of myself in this light and feel stronger and more confident as a result.

Am I completely recovered? I am considerably recovered. Gone is the wheelchair, the stick and the tin of Jersey Royals. I have, to some extent, forgotten how ill I was, but I am still continually grateful for the ability to sit on a dining chair. I drive, work, shop, socialize and go on holiday. I have had seven books published. I can't do what I used to do but - thinking about it - nobody can do what I used to do - and live. I still have to keep my stress levels down.

The way I see it: I tried to push my body to do more than was good for it. My body stopped me. It continues to stop me if I try to over-exert myself. I reckon it knows what it's doing. Although endowed with a tiny sparrow's body, I have the drive and determination of a wasp on speed. Given half a chance, I probably would over-do all over again. Maybe, if I hadn't got ME, I'd have got something worse. I am a workaholic. I say 'am' a workaholic because one can never be completely cured, just reformed. I see ME as a limiting mechanism to stop people like me doing themselves irreparable physical damage.

Some people can trek across the Sahara or cycle up the Pyrenees. Evidently, we are not one of them. But we are still capable of achieving great things – just not all this afternoon.

Most useful aid to recovery - a good bed

Recommended book - "Living with ME: The Chronic, Post-viral Fatigue Syndrome" by Dr Charles Shepherd

Recommended website - www.me-cfs-treatment.com (Dr David Smith's site)

Margaret's advice - once recovered don't neglect to idle

Margaret

Mike's Story

It was the doughnuts that did it

It was the doughnuts that did it. No kidding. Doughnuts on the way to work, coffee all day at my desk, bagels for lunch, pasta for dinner and cookies in front of the TV.

I was working in New Jersey for a financial firm. It wasn't that stressful a job, but I ran on adrenaline anyway. I hardly saw my family because I left before the kids were up in the morning, and returned home after they were in bed. I didn't have a problem with that. My career came first. I had to work hard to make partner. Weekends I couldn't relax. My wife was forever telling me to slow down, but I couldn't. I just didn't seem able to unwind.

One day I went to work like any other day. I grabbed my doughnut and coffee from a take-out on the way up to the office. In the lift I suddenly felt so exhausted that I could barely stand. By the time the lift reached my floor I was on my knees and couldn't get up. I was so weak I couldn't hold my cup of coffee. My eyes were closing and all I wanted to do was lie down on the floor and sleep.

That was the last day I worked for five years. I lost my job. I lost my house. I nearly lost my wife and kids.

The medics could find nothing wrong with me. Hey great. I am unable to walk, I am unable to think or talk coherently or even stay awake. I am in pain all over. I have all the symptoms you guys know all about – and the doc could find nothing wrong with me. Did I get depressed? You bet I did. So then the doc says I'm depressed. Yeah, no surprise, but *because* I'm in this awful state pal, *because* you don't believe me, *because* my life has stopped, *because* I feel so ill.

I spent a great deal of the money that we didn't have visiting different interns, getting bloods done, scans and trying to survive without an income. I did eventually get a diagnosis of CFS but hey, what was the difference? There was no treatment available anyway. We couldn't pay the bills and my wife had to return to work and resented it. I couldn't cope with the kids at home. We had to downsize our house and my wife had to do the move on her own because I was too sick to help.

This went on for four long years, during which time I got suicidally depressed and resentful of a family that prevented me from taking my own life. You don't do that to kids do you, but I sure as hell didn't want to face a future of feeling so ill every single day for the rest of my life. As far as I could tell, nobody recovered from CFS and I was in it for the long run.

I was the first person I knew who recovered.

So how did I do it? An Austrian doctor called Dr Wolfgang Lutz gets the credit. I read his book "Life Without Bread – How A Low Carbohydrate Diet Can Save Your Life". Forget the title which is off-putting and makes it sound like a diet book - it most definitely isn't! It is a medical book written for medics and for the lay person about the effects of excess carbohydrates (glucose) on our physiology. Dr Lutz believes that we have been eating too many refined carbohydrates in the western world over the last forty-odd years, which is why we are all getting sick with cancer, heart disease and so on. He outlines his experience, since the 1960s, of treating and reversing these illnesses with the more old-fashioned low carbohydrate diet. There is a particularly informative chapter on how excess glucose interferes with the mitochondria in our cells, which are responsible for producing energy. I read that book and was convinced that my junk food American diet had caused a breakdown in my body's ability to deal with the normal stresses of daily life.

I followed Dr Lutz's dietary guidelines and within a year I was fit enough to return to work. In two years I was fitter than I had been before I got sick. Not only that, but as a surprising bonus I experienced what I can only call an 'inner peace' for the first time in my life. I even stopped grinding my teeth in my sleep. For as long as I can remember I had been unable to relax, 'fidgety', on edge. I now know that was because I was living on adrenaline, as a result of the highly processed carbohydrate-based diet, sodas and caffeine, which were sending my blood sugar levels berserk.

I started eating butter and red meat and the fat on my (organic) chicken. It took a while to convince my wife. I had been brought up on a low fat diet and prided myself on being a young man who cared about his health and fitness. I had no idea that a low fat diet was depleting me of the hormones I needed to function properly. Nathan Pritikin's flawed study of the 1970s was responsible for that – thanks Nathan.*

So what is CFS? Well I don't know what is causing yours – but I guess mine was caused by the appalling diet that we all eat in this so-called 'civilised' world. Ever wondered why we are keeling over left, right and centre in the western world with CFS due to 'stress' when folks in Iraq aren't? Despite the fact that they live in permanent fear of being bombed the minute they step outside their front door? It's nothing to do with me having more stress in my office job than those guys in Iraq, and everything to do with the fact that I am less able to deal with stress than they are. And why is that? Because we eat a crap diet and they don't!

So – that was all six years ago and I have been fit and healthy and able to cope with all the stresses that life has thrown at me ever since. My marriage survived, though it nearly didn't, and my kids are growing up to be wonderful people, despite all the difficult times we had to go through. I returned to work in finance and continued to work very hard. I never went back to the man-made carbohydrate-based diet I lived on before I got sick; or the sodas, or the caffeine. As a result I grew stronger over time and have remained physically strong, emotionally balanced and with the continued 'inner peace' that I discovered when I learned how to 'turn off' the adrenaline by eating the right foods and balancing my blood sugar levels. I am happier and 100% fitter in my forties than I ever was in my twenties, and I expect to be for a long time to come.

Most useful aid to recovery - a low carbohydrate, high good fat and protein diet

Recommended books
"Life Without Bread – How a Low Carbohydrate diet Can Save Your Life" by Dr Wolfgang Lutz
"Dangerous Grains" by Dr James Braly

Recommended website - www.westonaprice.org/knowyourfats/skinny.html*

Mike's advice - check out your diet before you do anything else

Mike Roger

Joanna's Story

Maybe we can use the power of the mind to overcome our illness

Hello all! To those of you who don't know me I'm Joanna, twenty-six, from Kegworth. I had ME for seven years following a very vicious flu attack and numerous bouts of tonsillitis – that is, before I heard of Phil Parker and the Lightning Process -and got well!

I first became ill in 1999. My story is much the same as everyone else's. I became ill, and was dismissed by doctors until all tests confirmed I had nothing wrong with me, so it must be ME. I read all the books, paced myself and took things easy when I needed to. Every alternative treatment was investigated, tablets taken, tinctures swallowed, body massaged and manipulated, but I still had ME.

I managed to get myself well enough to go to university, but it took me five years to do a three-year degree and I didn't get the award I would have done if I was well. Then, after graduation, I crashed totally. I had been about 70% on the ME scale, but fell to 25-35%. The last eighteen months were hell - lots of pain, total exhaustion and no life.

Then I read about the Lightning Process on a forum and decided to give it a go. A trip to London would take everything out of me, but I'd tried everything else and if it got me 20% better it would be worth it. You could say that I was cautiously optimistic about the treatment, but very sceptical and in need of convincing!

On January 2ⁿᵈ Mum and I headed down to London. We stayed in a 'Bed and breakfast' in Crouch End, quite close to the clinic, and my wheelchair was with us too. Little did I realise, as Mum pushed me down the road for tea the night before the first session, that it would be the last time I'd use it!

The first session was two hours long and I was really surprised that I managed well with it. I found it hard to concentrate on the 'Neighbours' storyline, so concentrating for this length of time was incredible. Phil explained everything in an up-beat, energetic manner with a bit of swearing thrown in (very down-to-earth language!) and when he could see that I was starting to flag he asked if I wanted a break. We stopped for some water, but he quickly revived me with going into what to do and how to do it. It was amazing how energised I started to feel as the session wore on.

He explained the following: when you become ill your body produces adrenaline as part of the stress response cycle. This is normal. One of the natural effects of adrenaline is to suppress your immune system, and if these levels are high enough some of us become more ill, the physical stress of which increases our adrenaline levels further, spiralling you into ME. Imagine you're a cave man. You have a cut on your leg. You see a tiger in front of you. Your adrenaline kicks in for a 'fight or flight response' to save you. What it stops doing, at this time, is healing your leg. That can wait, because healing at this point in time would be a waste of your valuable resources, which are better used to help you escape from the tiger first and heal later. With ME our adrenaline levels are so all over the place that we can't heal and get over our initial illness.

The Lightning Process is a way of working through a variety of stages to decrease the adrenaline levels, and ultimately give you a life you love. We don't want to feel pain or tiredness, but every few minutes we are thinking, mostly unconsciously, "what hurts?" "am I tired?". We do this over three hundred times a day probably. Each time we run these mental processes we are strengthening and reaffirming neural pathways in our brains. By running the Lightning Process and looking for good health you can create new neural pathways and nerve routes so that adrenaline levels go down, the immune system and blood sugar levels and everything else that is upset rectifies itself, thereby ridding you of ME. This works on the theory that ME is basically a self-maintaining adrenaline overdrive cycle, which in turn causes immune system dysfunction, poor digestion, poor thyroid function, poor control of blood sugar and so on. These are the things that create all of our symptoms. By getting rid of these you no longer have ME.

After that first session we returned to the B&B. I realised that I needed a drink, so I darted through the traffic to cross the road and bought a bottle of water. I then went up the stairs to our room and then stopped. I just realised what I had done. Without pausing, pain or tiredness! That night we went out for tea and I walked about five hundred metres to a restaurant. Just one day before I had struggled with fifty metres!

The second session the following day was just one hour long. We went through some of my problem areas, like pain, and what to do when …. scenarios. After that session we went shopping to Brent Cross – for one and a quarter hours! On my feet! It was amazing. My feet were hurting, but I realised that I'd not really used them for years, so it wasn't too surprising! We went to visit a friend in London that night and again I walked a good distance. I also climbed the stairs to her third floor flat with no problems. It was feeling like the old Jo was back.

On the way home after the third session I started to get a headache. I ran through the process and controlled it and it went. This was really odd – how can a mental trick effect the body like that? I am still not sure how it does it, but I know that it has worked for me!

In December I had tried to return something to Asda. I got part way and ended up sitting on the floor. I had walked fifty yards and was so exhausted and in so much pain that I just collapsed. However, a few months later I went on a week's holiday to Tenerife, where I swam for ages in the sea, walked miles everyday, climbed up nettings, slid down fireman's poles and crossed rope bridges on an assault course and had a fantastic, wheelchair free, health-full time!

The Lightning Process really helped my sleep too and it is now deeper and I feel refreshed in the mornings. Also if I am anxious about something I stop it before the worry is really there. Then I coach my way out of a negative thought process and change it to a positive outlook and plan. I have always been terrified of flying, but I enjoyed the flights to and from my holiday. I didn't even mind take off, landing and turbulence, which used to scare me silly. I now have strategies I can use for all those job interviews I'm going to go for!

The Process has only been used to treat ME very recently. At first Phil just used it to help people with self-esteem issues and lack of confidence. Then he found that he could help people with physical problems, like recurrent neck/back problems and asthma. He decided to try it out on a colleague who had suffered from ME for some years and it worked. They tried a couple of other people they knew with ME and got the same positive outcome.

Phil has treated less than 500 people so far, but there is a wonderful success rate for those who have learned and used the process. He has also used it with pop stars, sports people, businessmen, even a guy who turned over millions each day on the stock market. It helps with everything really.

This treatment may not be for everyone as it does involve the expense of spending three days in London and the treatment itself is quite costly, but in my experience it has been well worth it. I have spent a great deal of money on many other treatments and therapies that have not worked. There are a few practitioners other than Phil who teach the Lightning Process dotted around the country too.

For any of you reading this who think "well, she couldn't have had ME in the first place" (you'd be amazed how many people have said this to me), well I had it confirmed by my GP, two hospital specialists and Raymond Perrin (osteopath) who used me in his PhD research and said I was a perfect specimen of ME on the scans. And for any of you who are thinking that I'm saying ME is all in the mind – I'm not. It is all in the brain. The huge majority of us have had masses of tests which all came back saying that we were 'normal' and 'healthy' when it was obvious that we weren't. Maybe our brains are sending the wrong messages around, hormone levels are haywire and we are stuck in a vicious cycle we are not even aware of.

In July 2006 I spent three months in Ghana working as a volunteer. I worked at a Football Academy, taught at an orphanage, did a few shifts at a major hospital and spent eight weeks working with a Premiership football team, Accra Great Olympics! It was an amazing experience, and one that I will never forget. At times, when I was up before first light to go to training, walked four miles there and back, taught a mathematics and an English lesson, been for a swim, sorted out all the injuries at evening training and then been out dancing until four in the morning, I would suddenly get a bit emotional. How was I able to do so much, after seven years of being able to do so little? I appreciated the whole experience from a different angle - as well as the difference between the rich western world and the poverty of Africa, I could see and feel the difference between health and the lack of it, from a particularly personal view.

Since then I have been working. Nine months as a super temp, starting in the very busy Human Resources department of a training company, and then moving to recruitment. At the same time I was working in a gym. Most recently I have been working for a premiership rugby team, looking after up to ninety, eight to sixteen year old rugby playing kids, each week, as they are put through their paces. I have regained a great deal of confidence in my Sports Rehabilitation knowledge, despite the break that ME imposed on my career path. I have also made a number of contacts who will hopefully be able to help me on the next step.

Another big thing has been rejoining a theatre company. Whilst working full time I also rehearsed and was in a musical, "Sweet Charity", which was on for five nights. I loved every second of it and, yes, I did get tired, but so did everyone else! I had a blast and attended every after-show do. I have also just been in a concert and sang a few solos, something I hadn't done since the year before I got ill. It was terrifying, but I did it! I used all that I had learned through the Lightning Process and it got me through - although I was still shaking a bit.

So if you've just read this and thought "wow, that sounds really quite cool", then just get out there and try new treatments, especially the Lightning Process, and *know* that there is light at the end of the tunnel. Good luck to you all. I know what ME is like and I know that it is pure hell. There are times when you feel like giving up, crawling into your bed and not getting out. There are times when you have no choice but to do that. But have some hope that you can get better. If you can walk over white-hot coals and the skin on your feet doesn't burn, maybe you can use the power of the mind to overcome your illness. I know that I have!

Most useful aid to recovery - The Lightning Process

Recommended websites
www.philparker.org
www.lightningprocess.com

Joanna

Maureen's Story

Big Cracks

One day I woke up and couldn't get out of bed. It wasn't as sudden as it sounds…it had been coming for a long time. It felt almost like small cracks in the sidewalk that over time, with harsh weather and foot traffic, became big cracks. I could see the small cracks growing, the periodic exhaustion, the achy joints, the unexplainable rashes, benign tumours and constant colds. I knew something was wrong, but I didn't know how wrong it was.

It was on my thirty-fifth birthday that I knew something had finally broken. I couldn't get my body temperature right – I went from sweating to shivering. My mind was foggy and I couldn't seem to concentrate. I was exhausted from almost a year of insomnia and was fighting just to get through the day. And then there was the sore throat I had been battling for two months…

I had something similar seven years previously, but not as severe. It was like a severe cold in my chest, an extreme ache and exhaustion, coupled with a lack of mental focus. It started after a trip to San Francisco where I caught a cold and never seemed to recover. After a year of doctors throwing their hands up, one finally gave me steroid packs and it magically went away.

The difference this time was that on my birthday the crack became a huge crack and by the end of the party I could barely stand. The next couple of weeks I kept telling myself it was just the flu. By September I felt I was well enough to go to New York to meet a friend with whom I had promised we'd hit the town. The first day I seemed fine, but by the second day I couldn't get out of bed. I stayed in bed the entire day but made it out that night and got drunk just to stay awake with my friend. By the third day, I was forced to leave New York and go back home because I could no longer function. When I arrived home I got into bed and didn't get up again for over a month.

I had CFS. The hard thing about CFS is that no one takes you seriously. First of all, it is not something tangible like cancer which everyone understands. Many people thought I was just depressed or tired. I think the name 'chronic fatigue syndrome' is also an unfortunate term. It doesn't sound credible and has been deemed 'The Yuppy Disease', so that makes it even harder for others to grasp.

The distressing part was that everything I read said that there was no cure. I went into a deep depression for a period, thinking that there may be no hope. One day I realised that if I didn't adjust my mental outlook I would go into a black hole I may not be able to escape from. I couldn't let myself go there. I decided that my only focus every day was to find a way to get better. I began to do some research online and soon came across information about Dr Jacob Teitelbaum.

Dr Teitelbaum is a doctor in Maryland who has great success treating CFS sufferers and who himself had CFS as a medical student. I called his office and set up an appointment to fly to Maryland and he ordered lots of blood tests for me. He was the first doctor who had done blood work and I finally felt like someone was taking me seriously. When my tests came back it showed that many of the systems that controlled my body were out of balance, including my adrenal gland and thyroid.

I went on Dr. Teitelbaum's regime of diet, vitamins and herbs and some pharmaceutical medicines. (They are outlined in his book, "From Fatigued to Fantastic"). The first couple of months were hard and I almost gave up. But slowly the fog started to lift. Each day I would go to the beach and walk as far as I could. At first it was only ten feet. Soon it was more. Then I was walking fast. Next I was running.

I now have more sustainable energy that I ever did before my experience with CFS and my life has been better than it ever was before. I have travelled frequently, to Brazil, Africa, Aspen, New York and New Mexico in the past year, and have many more trips planned. Because I am not as cranky as I was previously due to fatigue, it is easier for me to maintain relationships and nuture them. My CFS experience taught me so much. I can now really enjoy everything, because I have a new perspective on life and health.

During my illness I also found acupuncture, meditation and rolfing incredibly important. I still receive acupuncture twice a week, meditate daily and have a periodic rolfing session - and will continue this for the rest of my life. (Rolfing is a form of hands on, connective tissue manipulation).

Chronic Fatigue is a devastating disease, not only for the patient but for their loved ones as well. But don't let anyone tell you there is no hope - keep your spirit alive and, with the right treatment, your body will follow.

Most useful aid to recovery - Dr Jacob Teitelbaum

Recommended website - www.endfatigue.com

Maureen's advice - listen to what **yo**ur gut is telling you. Explore alternative options as well as western medicine. Change your diet – food makes an enormous difference. Don't let your spirit go – keep believing there is a way to get better. Don't bottle up your emotions. Also, during my bout with CFS I made a conscious decision never to think of myself as a sick person. I just decided that this was a temporary thing that I could beat. I know it sounds crazy, but by not defining myself by CFS I was able to stay positive and get healthy.

Maureen

Rob's Story

Miracles can happen

Until late September 1992, our son was just like any other boy of thirteen. He was happily settled in his secondary school, had his own paper round, good friends and had just managed to climb Snowdon. Life was good.

It was after having a really enjoyable time celebrating his friend's birthday that life changed. At first it seemed as if Robert had a very heavy cold which made him feel ill enough to spend a while in bed, suffering from really bad headaches and sleep disturbance. However it was when Robert was walking around that we noticed he was unable to walk properly, his pace was slow and he resembled an old person staggering around. We alerted our GP and Robert began weekly blood tests. We were never told what he was being tested for - it was best not to know. All the test results were negative.

A month into the illness Robert was admitted to our local hospital for tests. At the end of the two-day stay we were told Robert was suffering from post viral fatigue. Robert came home, but he had picked up a particularly nasty gastric virus, which weakened him considerably and his condition worsened.

At the beginning of December the next step was a meeting with a psychiatrist. To reach the appropriate psychiatrist's room my husband had to carry Robert up two flights of stairs as there were no facilities for disabled people. The interview went well and Robert, although exhausted from all the travelling, was able to answer questions appropriately, proving that he didn't have a psychiatric problem. The psychiatrist set up hydrotherapy and school sessions at a local hospital to begin in the New Year.

By December 17th Robert could no longer walk, feed himself, or chew food. He was completely dependent on us. He suffered from cracking headaches and had to live in a darkened room because he couldn't stand the light.

The New Year came and the ambulance picked us up for hydrotherapy. Once Robert was on a seat in the ambulance he had to lean against me, as he was now unable to sit up by himself. It was a major effort to get Robert into the water and out again, and as you can imagine, he was totally exhausted afterwards and had to face the unknown prospect of school.

Before school began there was a long lunch break and we had arrived at the beginning of it. There was no bed available so I made Robert as comfortable as possible and we waited for school to begin. School was supposed to be an educational and social experience. Robert was wheeled in front of a computer screen and given games to play. Three minutes were enough – he couldn't stand the brightness of the screen, and his hands, which he was now unable to write with, were unable to operate the computer keys for any longer. All Robert wanted to do was get home and rest, but we had to wait at the hospital for the late afternoon transport.

By the time we eventually got home Robert was in a terrible state, so I cancelled school and we carried on with hydrotherapy twice a week. Life was hard for Robert, every time he had hydrotherapy he spent days attempting to recover the energy he had used and then it was time for the next session. One morning after my husband had carried Robert downstairs and helped him to dress in readiness for transport to hydrotherapy no ambulance arrived. We waited an hour only to be told hydrotherapy had finished. Although it was a very annoying situation, it was also a relief because hydrotherapy had not helped Robert at all

– in fact it had set him back. Throughout the month of hydrotherapy no one had checked on Robert's progress.

It was about this time we met John, Robert's Home Tutor. John was like a breath of fresh air coming into a situation where positive help was needed, and he provided it by keeping Robert going educationally. It's not easy teaching someone who is bed bound, there are definite limitations, but John was excellent and his efforts helped Robert tremendously.

Before I go any further I must mention our own version of J.M. Barrie's 'Nana' in Peter Pan – ours was feline not canine. Lacey came to us before Robert's illness began, a mature cat with a pronounced limp causing the other cats to be wary of her and respond physically to her foul language. So Lacey decided to become an indoor cat. When Robert became severely disabled Lacey eased herself into the role of constant companion, making sure Robert was only alone at night. Doctors' visits and home tuition didn't bother Lacey; she had found that her love of human company had led her into the role of feline carer.

Our General Practitioner was lovely but never used the name for the illness and was continually looking for another reason for the strange symptoms that had created a halt in Robert's teenage life.

Our next visit was to a neurologist who gave Robert a thorough and exhausting check over. Then our GP, the psychiatrist and neurologist got together and devised a rehabilitation plan for Robert. We met with them and they explained that Robert would be admitted to our local Hospital, where he would undergo physiotherapy and schooling and not be allowed out until he could walk. A bed was found the following Monday, so we took him in, handed him over to the nurses and left him. We were given strict instructions not to visit during the day. My husband went in that evening to visit Robert and came back saying Robert was in a terrible state.

The next morning I knew that as soon as I had got our three younger children to school I had to get to the hospital. So I defied the doctors and headed off to the hospital. By the time I arrived it was lunchtime and what I saw was alarming. I had a strong feeling that all was not well and it certainly wasn't. As soon as I got to the ward I saw Robert in a terrible state, having been totally drained of every ounce of his limited energy through physiotherapy and schooling, being wheeled back to bed. He hadn't been dressed, had breakfast or been to the loo, because at this stage in his illness he needed help to look after himself and he didn't want a nurse to help him. I don't know what would have happened if I hadn't turned up when I did.

I was able to sort Robert out as best as I could, but then I had to go and pick the children up from school before returning with them to the hospital. I phoned my husband to explain the situation and we agreed there and then that enough was enough and that this sort of treatment was going to have serious consequences for Robert if we didn't act quickly. We could see our son slipping into a far worse state than he was already in. So we all met up at the hospital and waited for the doctor to come round, and told him that Robert's stay in the hospital was history.

That night Robert was home again and we decided not to accept any more treatment unless we knew it wouldn't have an adverse effect. It took Robert weeks to get back to where he was before his visit to the hospital. (I must add at this point that Robert's younger brother had been beautifully cared for at the same hospital for the last six weeks of his very short life.) So life went on and we took it a day at a time, never knowing whether we would ever get our son back. No one could predict the outcome of Robert's illness.

Each year we managed a family holiday. Whether this was a good idea for Robert was debatable, but the family had to carry on as normally as possible and it was important for the rest of the children to get away. Our first holiday was Butlins where we could hire a wheelchair for Robert. Then we went to Spain where we thought the heat might help Robert. It was in 1995 that we discovered Thornley House and spent several holidays there, making new friends. Robert had his own feline carer who kept him company when he was too ill to leave his bedroom. Nothing was too much at Thornley House. It is a Hotel that caters for the elderly and disabled, so agreeing to take in us six was quite an undertaking, but they did it and it was marvellous. We will always be grateful to them for their help in our time of need. We have been back many times and the staff are wonderful.

At this point I have to mention friends, who are so important at times like these. Thank you Ian, Aaron and Trevor, for helping Robert through his illness. Life would have been so much harder without your continual visits, phone calls and understanding.

By December 1993 Robert still had no official medical diagnosis. Ironically we knew what this horrendous condition was that was robbing our son of a normal life, and had done since a month into the illness, but we had been unable to find a medical professional in Oxfordshire who understood ME. We had heard about a Dr Alan Franklin in Chelmsford, so our health authority paid for us to go out of the county for an appointment with him. What a wonderful relief that was, to meet someone who believed in our son and was prepared to admit he was suffering from ME. Although we'd have given anything not to have Robert in this state, he was and here was someone who could understand and accept the illness. It was such a relief. My own personal description of Dr Franklin would be Christ-like. He was wonderful and although he was unable to give us a miracle cure, he gave us confidence and a sense of not being alone as we battled on. So nearly fifteen months into the illness we had the diagnosis of ME. At last someone from the medical side believed in our son and this was extremely important.

Life carried on and we came into contact with a lot of wonderful people who remembered to ask how Robert was each time they saw us and prayed for him over the years. Dr Parkin and his lovely daughter came all the way from Lincolnshire to try electro-acupuncture on Robert, but unfortunately it only made Robert very sleepy.

Just around the time Robert was sixteen he was admitted to Birmingham Children's Hospital because our GP was still puzzled by Robert's condition and wanted to make sure that there was nothing else medically wrong. Luckily my husband was in between jobs at the time and was able to stay in the hospital with Robert to assist with personal care. During the next two weeks Robert had a thorough M.O.T. The children and I visited mid-week and Robert came home at the weekend. The hospital staff on the children's ward were extremely kind to Robert, but as time went on we began to feel that pressure was being put on us to allow Robert to be admitted to another ward, where he would stay until he walked again and we would only be allowed to visit a couple of times a week. All this sounded very familiar.

Luckily I had a contact with a daughter on this ward so I was able to find out a bit about it. I also managed to visit the locked ward, which was beautifully furnished and found out it had a mixture of youngsters, some with ME, and others with psychiatric problems. I was able to talk to Robert about possible admission to the ward and we made the decision not to go ahead with it. All Robert's tests were fine, so we took him home believing that family, friends, pets and home life was far more important than being locked up on a ward miles away.

In September Robert began to attend college. West Oxfordshire College welcomed Robert on to a Foundation Course where they were wonderful to him. Ross became his personal tutor and George became Robert's regular taxi driver. Robert enjoyed talking to George on the way to college. Other special people played a part in supporting Robert. He needed a lot of help being in a wheelchair and unable to do much for himself. He would return from a short session at college absolutely exhausted and need two days of complete rest to enable him to build up his limited strength for the next session. However, somehow he coped with it and managed to finish the Foundation Course and go on to get two GCSEs. He also attempted a maths A-level, but had to give it up. It was impossible with the severity of his ME. Robert was also unable write at this point so he had to use a scribe.

Whilst Robert was doing his College courses, we moved to a new house. Robert was able to be downstairs all the time and he was able to have a change of doctor - someone who believed in ME. These factors made life easier for all of us.

We'd had contact with lots of physiotherapists, each one working with Robert as she thought best. But treating someone with ME isn't easy and only one had really understood the situation - until we found Kathy. Kathy was an absolute treasure, she worked at Robert's pace, had a sense of humour that matched his, and we looked forward to her weekly visits. Kathy began to work very gently with Robert in 1999 and towards the end of that year we began to notice that things were happening. The cracking headaches began to recede; I wasn't buying weekly supplies of Hedex Extra. We became aware that for the first time since the beginning of Robert's illness he could tolerate the light, his bedroom curtains were open during the day. He began to recover the strength in his hands and gradually he regained the ability to write. This was a marvellous happening. It was lovely to see Robert using a pen again after all this time, writing cheques, cards and letters without us doing it for him. His writing was exactly as it had been seven years ago, before this awful illness happened.

Christmas came and went and life for Robert was a bit better. He was still unable to walk and needed a lot of care, but his hands were able to write again and that was a major development. Then came one of the most memorable days of our lives. March 2nd 2000. Kathy arrived, and with her came a pair of crutches. We had no idea of Kathy's plans. She hadn't told Robert he was going to attempt to stand up, but he did. He managed to stand up for forty seconds. It wasn't until after Kathy had gone that reality hit us. This was it, the beginning of something amazing. Robert being able to walk again. Words can't express the emotions of that day.

Each day of the following week Robert stood up with his crutches and we had to time him. He would have one attempt and then a rest followed by another attempt, his standing time gradually increasing daily. Kathy moved Robert on to stepping backwards and forward and he practised this for a week. A very short walk followed this from one room to another. Robert's progress was rapid and he very quickly moved on from crutches to a stick to walking independently. It was marvellous to see him walk down the garden or climb the stairs.

Kathy had a wonderful surprise when Robert was sitting at the top of the stairs waiting for her to arrive on one of her visits. As soon as Robert became confident enough to visit Kathy at the hospital, home visits finished. Of all the people who came into Robert's life throughout his illness, Kathy will be one of the people we will always be extremely grateful to.

By 2002 Robert was leading an almost normal life. He completed two AS levels and applied for university the following year. Progress was rapid. During that summer we went back to Thornley House, Devon. We decided to climb Hay Tor, the highest peak on Dartmoor. We didn't know if Robert could manage it, but he was determined to try. It was a real achievement for Robert to reach the summit. He had needed a few rest stops on the way up, but still managed to beat the family with two small children to the top. Everybody at Thornley house was delighted. James, the owner said, "When I first met you, Robert, in 1995, you couldn't lift your head off the pillow". Miracles can happen.

Diane Fairfield

Postscript by Rob

I was more scared by that first month of recovery than I have ever been

Looking back on my illness now, six years after recovering, it seems like a different person's life. I remember my life during the illness and I remember how quickly time passed. It seems strange to say that, but I got into a daily routine that rarely changed. I'd wake up, eat breakfast, rest for a few hours, eat lunch, rest for a few hours, eat dinner, rest for a few hours, then go to sleep. That was the pattern each and every day, and so much time just slipped by.

I would listen to speech radio occasionally or watch a little bit of television. I forgot what it was like to be well. I forgot what my old life was like and I couldn't imagine being well. My sisters and brother were going through school and teenage experiences and telling me about it, but I couldn't visualise myself in their situation.

My life was my bedroom and my routine. I remember thinking about riding my bike and how happy that made me feel, how I used to enjoy cycling through the woods and fields with friends and how much I would like to do that again. I never doubted that I would recover, but I didn't know how it was going to happen. Would it be a sudden transition over a period of days, or a gradual process? What would it be like to tell people that I was better, how would they react?

As it happened, I think my recovery was almost as rapid as my descent into illness. It only took about a month to go from being bed bound to walking unaided. I gradually started to notice that I was not getting so tired from activities. Then I stopped feeling tired all the time, and found I was able to do more physiotherapy. After a few weeks I was able to stand, and then to walk again.

People were so happy for me. Friends were thrilled, family members cried, it was a really emotional time. Everyone was happy and I wanted to be happy, but inside I was scared. I had not expected to be gripped by fear, but I was more scared for that first month of recovery than I have ever been. My life was thrown into a state of flux. I suddenly had a future that I had not prepared for, and no idea how I was going to build a life. I had an overwhelming sense that I had been left behind by everyone else. My school peers' lives had been a constantly ascending slope of development and achievement, whilst my own life had been on a plateau during my illness, and now they were unreachable.

Gradually, with the support of my family and friends, I adjusted to my new life and taking little steps into the outside world I became a normal person again. I went on a bus to my local town for physiotherapy and went to a pub with a friend. By small increments, my life became comparable to that of other people's. The fear subsided to a degree.

When I initially enrolled at college I wanted to do five A-levels, just to catch up as quickly as possible. Fortunately I was talked out of this, and settled for two! I was worried about being older than the other students, because I was twenty-two at this point and all the other A-level students were sixteen years old and fresh from school. But it was not an issue. I made a lot of friends and fitted in easily. My age was not a problem, and I don't think many of them guessed that I was older, or that I had been ill. I certainly didn't bring it up in conversation. These students became my peers, and I found that I had a life like them. I socialised with them and they shared their interests and taste in music and film with me. This was when I started to feel happy. It didn't matter that I had been ill. I was picking up my life and fitting into a new social group.

When I got to university, I found that there were a number of mature students on my course and this was a great comfort. I shared a house with four other students and found that I was no longer unique or different. A number of the other mature students had needed to change direction in life or had experienced some traumatic setback. I gradually found out about some of my old classmates from school and found that few of them were any further ahead in life than I was. I discovered that the ideal life I imagined many of them to be leading just didn't exist.

Everyone has problems and obstacles to over come, you just don't let them beat you down. Imagine the life you want, and work out how to achieve it. Plan for the future. In many ways it was an advantage to have a fresh start in life. I suspect that had I stayed at school I would probably have done badly in my exams because I was not really interested in studying. I would probably be in a bad job now if I had not left school through illness!

Thankfully I am physically fit and have not suffered any relapses since recovering. I was even able to work for two months as a labourer on a building site a couple of summers ago. I carried bricks and bags of cement and was breaking concrete all day, five days a week, without any problems at all.

As it turned out, my life is great now and I am enjoying it thoroughly. After having graduated from Oxford Brookes University with a First Class Honours Degree in Architecture, I moved to London to work in a large Architectural Practice. I am happy to say that I live a perfectly normal life.

Most useful aid to recovery - regular half-hour periods of complete rest in bed with no television, music or radio and with the phone off the hook.

Rob's advice - believe you will get better. It may take a while, but it *will* happen. Only consult a doctor who believes in ME. It is so much easier. Some doctors can do far more harm than good. Make sure you are resting properly with no distractions, in a quiet and relaxing environment, and try not to think about anything stressful. I was not resting properly in the first few years of my illness and I suffered for it. Don't worry about being left behind by other people, time is not important, nor is age; it doesn't take long to pick your life up again. Don't forget how fantastic the world outside your house is. Remember happy times. Forget the bad, they will not exist when you recover. Keep pacing yourself when you do recover. Don't have a hectic life. Focus on the most important aspects and donate your energy to these. The rest can be picked up when you have the energy.

Rob Fairfield

Barbara's story

At seventy one I have more energy than I had at forty

At the age of seventy-one I have more energy than I had at forty. At forty I was a teacher. I had two children, a husband and a home to look after and I found it all very tiring. I couldn't keep on top of the housework. I found it an effort to go out with my husband or have friends around for dinner, so these things didn't happen and we led a very quiet life. I often suffered from bouts of feeling completely drained. For example, shopping for school uniform would leave me shattered for days afterwards. I always enjoyed painting and sewing but I lost interest in these activities. I also stopped reading and having intelligent conversation as I didn't seem able function at that level anymore. Every time I went to the doctor complaining of feeling tired and down, he said it was due to my hormones – pre-menopause, menopause, and later post-menopause.

At fifty I took early retirement. I hoped that this would give me a new lease of life, but instead I just collapsed in a heap. Getting up and dressed in the morning took every ounce of willpower and energy that I had. My marriage, my relationships with my children, my family and my friends all suffered for my poor health. I wasn't a fun person to be around. I was always irritable with the children. I became indecisive and anxious. I was always tired, always 'down'. I avoided anything that required effort. Meals became simple affairs or didn't happen at all. I wanted to live on my own so I didn't have to feel guilty about being a bad wife and mother; so that I didn't have to get up and cope with the family, so that I could take to my bed and stay there forever if I wanted to, without impacting on anyone else.

By the age of sixty my world had become smaller and smaller. I think eventually I couldn't remember what it felt like to be well and out there in the big wide world. I led a greatly reduced, quiet, uneventful life. Any 'events' emotional or physical, left me feeling drained for days afterwards. I didn't deal with even minor stresses at all well and often felt very down without understanding why.

Of course I did try to get well. I didn't just sit around for twenty-five years. I did the rounds of the NHS consultants, getting my diagnosis of ME along the way. I didn't try the alternative therapies that everyone tries today, my doctor didn't believe in them, but I did see a psychiatrist who pronounced me of sound mind. To be honest, by the age of sixty I had given up hope of ever being well. I had learned to live within the four walls of my house and again, if I'm being honest about it, it was now much easier to remain there. Just like a fly caught in a spider's web I discovered that the more I struggled the worse I got. So I sat there and waited to die.

One day, my daughter rang me up. She had just returned from a lecture by Nancy Appleton PhD. Dr Appleton is a nutritionist and lecturer in the USA who warns against the horrors of sugar. My daughter enthusiastically declared that she would cut sugar out of her diet completely, sure that her irritable bowel syndrome, which she had had since a teenager, would be cured. She recommended strongly that I cut out my afternoon tea and biscuits, toast and marmalade and all other foods that I consider essential to my happiness. I wasn't too amused. After all, I had little enough pleasure in my life and food seemed a harmless one to me. So I humoured her, but did nothing about it. Every time she rang I said, yes darling, I *will* do something about it, I promise.

One day, she sent me a book by Dr Appleton called "Lick the Sugar Habit". I read it as I ate my toast and marmalade. I didn't want to do anything about my diet, but by then my daughter's irritable bowel syndrome had resolved and I realised that I was never going to get her off my back until I gave it a go. I agreed to a three month trial. This was the first time I went against my doctor's advise, which was to stick to the 'normal' diet that I was eating and not to try any 'crazy' diets.

Gamely I gave it my all. My daughter devised a new 'diet' for me. She cut out my beloved morning toast and marmalade. No more afternoon biscuits. Not even any bread for sandwiches! I was not about to start cooking complicated meals so she wrote me a very easy plan. I was allowed to eat a German breakfast of cheese and ham with fruit; bacon and eggs was also allowed if my husband was kind enough to cook it for me. I used packet salads and tubs of coleslaw and potato salad and cold meats and cheeses and eggs or tuna for an easy lunch. And dinner would be the traditional meat and two vegetables. Evenings before bed I had a whey protein milkshake drink from a large tub with a picture of a man's chest with massive muscles on it.

I promised three months – and that was five years ago. I don't want you to think it was easy. It wasn't. I have struggled. Goodness how I have struggled to do what seems to be such a simple thing as cut sugar out of my diet. Of course, it isn't just 'sugar', don't be fooled, cutting out sugar means cutting out anything that *turns* into sugar (glucose) in your bloodstream – so that means lots of other nice things too. But goodness gracious me, it was worth it, because after about two months I began to wake up more easily in the mornings. I began to feel naturally more cheerful. My head felt clearer and less 'foggy'. I found that my stamina increased, my energy was slowly returning and I was able to do things that I hadn't done for a long time, like reading intelligent books for example and planting daffodils in the garden.

Of course it wasn't a dramatic recovery. It was very slow. In fact, I think it took about two years for me to start living what you would call a 'normal' life again. And it wasn't a steady improvement all the time. I found it hard to stick to the diet and was forever falling off the bandwagon. It felt like two steps forward and one step backward. I thought that I would never have the self-control to stay off sugar forever. And indeed I haven't. But keeping off it for most of the time has enabled me to regain a life worth living and the energy to enjoy it.

It seems to me that sugar really is the white poison that Professor Yudkin, Professor of Nutrition at London University, called it in his book "Pure, White and Deadly" in the 1970s. It seems to me that too much of that pure, white and deadly sugar has been responsible for a less than joyous life for me. I have no doubt that had I lived a hundred years previously that I would have been in very good health – unless of course I had died in childbirth instead.

So, my daughter has been free of irritable bowel syndrome thanks to Dr Appleton's visit to the UK – and I have regained a life I never thought to enjoy again. At seventy-one I have more energy that I had at forty. Toast and marmalade, caffeine, breakfast cereal and afternoon biscuits are a thing of the past - as is my ME – and thank heaven for that!

Most useful aid to recovery - Cutting out sugar, flour, caffeine and *all* processed food

Recommended books
"Lick the Sugar Habit" by Nancy Appleton PhD
"Pure, White and Deadly: Problem of Sugar" by John S Yudkin
"The Sugar Blues" by William Duffy

Recommended website - www.nancyappleton.com

Barbara's advice - Don't waste twenty-five years of your life as I did, eating all your favourite foods but not realising how much they are contributing to your poor health. And don't waste your time worrying about your worries - when you are feeling better they will either vanish, or you will be able to deal with them.

Barbara Rivers

Ian's Story

My cure occurred in an instant

There can be no doubt that my cure was due to a certain kind of treatment, because it occurred in an instant, during my first session with the therapist. I'm not saying this in hindsight - I realised it at the time. It's almost an embarrassment to me, now that I have trained in the same therapy, to realise that my own cure was quite unorthodox, yet not unique. You might not believe me, yet what can I do but tell it the way it was?

So where to start? Believe it or not, this is around my fifth attempt to tell the story. I have abandoned the others because they are too much like autobiographical memoirs. They set the context of my family, personal life, spiritual state and so on. Some versions were sad, reflecting on how many years of my life were wasted in the misery and frustration of ME. Others were more upbeat, reflecting on how much I learned from the illness and subsequent recovery. In this instance, I'll try and keep to a single topic: how I got well.

First, did I really have ME and how long for? My symptoms go back to 1974, when I was struck down with some mystery illness. My limbs became so heavy I could hardly walk. I had been exposed to a form of hepatitis and it seemed that my liver function was down. I had tests over the years which showed I was normal, so it seemed strange that sometimes I felt so weak and tired, with a variety of other unpleasant symptoms.

In 1992 I was given an exclusion diagnosis of ME by Dr Weir at the Royal Free Hospital in Coppetts Wood, North London. Very slowly, my health got worse over the next fifteen years. Up till 1998 I was able to work full-time, but travelling to get there became an increasing problem and I had to confess my limitations to bosses. I was then forced to work part-time or did small contracts and commissions at home.

Overall, I tried to pace myself and my relapses always seemed due to miscalculation or emergency. I learned pacing from a telephone support person recommended by the ME Association. I used to ring her up as a kind of agony aunt. She published a book on ME later on, but I think in retrospect that her advice was more hindrance than help.

Pacing for me involved an ever-diminishing scope of activity, with use of a wheelchair eventually, for any outings that involved more than driving myself from door to door. I was dependent on others for shopping, cooking and so forth and feared I would never get better. I am tempted to illustrate how I coped and didn't cope by telling you a lot more. It might be interesting but would be irrelevant. Suffice to say that I made a number of adjustments and simplifications, in both worldly and spiritual life. I moved some way in the direction of wisdom, happiness and fulfilment. So why was I still plagued with this chronic fatigue thing? What lesson was it still trying to teach me?

One morning I raged against it with the fiery strength of a lion caught in a trap by hunters. That was the moment I sent out my passionate cry for help. In fury, I typed in something like 'ME/CFS waited long enough for cure', as if sending a complaining telegram to God rather than just entering keywords into Google. I immediately hit on David Mickel's book, 'Chronic Fatigue Syndrome, ME and Fibromyalgia – The Long Awaited Cure'. Had my cry been heard? I made an appointment with a local practitioner, Alistair, who lived a few miles away. He sounded very confident.

When I arrived for the first session he explained that it would take one and a half hours, to allow time for history-taking as well as treatment. I tried to tell him as much as I could, answering the anticipated questions before he asked them and messing up the structure he'd planned. This was partly due to a strange sense of impatience.

He explained the theory and said I would have to keep a journal, which we would dissect in our next session in two weeks' time. I was thinking, "I've waited so terribly, terribly long. I am sure this is what I have waited for. Give it to me now! How can I wait two weeks for the next instalment?" I felt as a mother would feel when giving birth, with the baby's head already engaged, if the midwife suggested completing the delivery on a future date! I rudely interrupted Alastair and asked him whether the therapy offered instant or gradual cure. He replied that it could be instant, though whether someone could cope with that was another matter.

This was the turning point. He explained that my symptoms were not caused by exertion but by an internal alarm system, which in CFS never gets switched off. I recognised that this was right, from some of the symptoms I used to experience.

Suddenly, something happened inside me that felt neither mental nor physical. Suppose you've been lying half-awake in the night, disturbed for hours by the racket of someone's burglar alarm. You almost get used to its rhythm. You adjust to it and drift off back to sleep. Then suddenly it stops. You wonder what happened. Silence sounds strange. That's just a metaphor, but it felt a bit like that, right there in the session. It was dramatic and it conveyed to me a profound knowledge that I was cured. It happened near the end of the session and I didn't say anything to Alastair. But here is an email, unedited, which I sent him a week later:

"Dear Alastair

I am so glad I asked you if the therapy can work instantaneously, because I let it do that and it did. As soon as I walked out of the consulting room I knew. It is as if a switch was thrown and the light bulb was illuminated.

I wanted to write and tell you the same day, but caution dictated that I should wait a while. And so now it has been a week and the certainty, the deep knowledge, has not wavered. I have done more physically, but the main thing I have done is rejoice in my new freedom, my recovered abilities and the sheer wonder and joy of a miracle. The fact that there is an explanation does not diminish the sense of miracle.

All week I have been fine. Aches, certainly, the symptoms try to grab me at times and persuade me that all is not well, but my deep knowledge - that is what I call it - has so far remained intact and I see no reason why it should not gain in assurance every day.

So I will say that the cure was instantaneous, but adjusting to it physically and mentally is something I am happy to take time over and savour.

Thank you for presenting to me what I needed to know so effectively. I will see you for the next session as agreed.

Best regards, Ian"

His response, also unedited here, was more cautious ....

"Dear Ian

I'm totally delighted with your clarity. Also to hear that you have got a firewall up against the viruses of doubt and uncertainty. Things can happen. Sometimes dealing with one level opens up another. Sometimes to test you three things happen on one day. Even if this brings on a temporary blip, know that once you have found the exit route you need never get lost again.

I look forward to our next meeting. Alastair."

In our second meeting he continued to be cautious. He told me off for not having kept a journal. We analysed a small incident in which I had felt the old symptoms, even though they cleared up unusually fast.

He proposed a further appointment but I said I would call him as and when I felt the need. I never did. I was now equipped to understand myself and knew what to do. There have been times when old symptoms have bothered me a little, but I've known they were flashbacks and not the real thing.

One year on, I am possibly fitter, at sixty-four, than I've been in my whole life.

My recovery happened in a single conscious moment and the rest has just been getting used to it. There has been a recovery of stamina and confidence, also a process of reconnection with my whole earlier life, at all ages. Before I got ill, walking had been one of my favourite recreations, and one of the greatest joys has been to discover country footpaths, examining nature closely as the seasons change, taking photos and sketching with pastels. I can now do whatever I want, and life holds the same excitement each day as for an adventurous child.

If I wanted I could live as I lived before, but I'm making better choices than that. The therapy has taught me to be guided by my deep body-wisdom, and let 'head' be a servant. This works very well! Everything falls into place. Though the experience of ME seemed so miserable and chronic and imprisoning at the time, looking back I have no regrets. The illness did what it was meant to do: stop me in my tracks and make me realign my life. I don't think about 'lost time'; but if it was lost, I am certainly making up for it now, and since my own recovery I have had the privilege of seeing others do the same.

Most useful aid to recovery - Mickel Therapy

Recommended website - www.mickeltherapy.com

Ian

Tracey's Story

The dirtier you are the more fun you've had

When I was twenty-three life was pretty good! I lived with my (then) partner and our dog and had a great job working for a large telecommunications company as a Trainer. Looking back, my life was busy. I had a very active social life, I was ambitious, I loved my job and I often worked very long days. I went to the gym regularly, enjoyed long walks in the countryside and was fit and healthy. I was a very lively and bubbly person, intelligent and alert, always on the go and known for being quite excitable. I really enjoyed having fun and was often described as "always smiling" or "here comes trouble". In a nice way, I hope!

I had worked in Birmingham city centre in telecommunications for just over a year. I thoroughly enjoyed it and worked with a really nice group of people who were friends as well as colleagues. We worked long hours, sometimes twelve hours a day and often went to a wine bar after work to wind down. On Friday of each week this would stretch into a night out, going to bars and clubs and finishing the week off with a stress-busting bang!

At home my partner and I had bought a run-down house and were doing lots of work on it to make it a home. We had a dog which we took for long walks and we enjoyed going on day trips and holidays. I had a large network of friends who would pop round and with whom

I would go shopping or for coffee. I can honestly say that at the time I was pretty satisfied with my lot in life.

During April 1995 work was particularly busy, as it was at this time every year, and I was in long meetings every day. At the end of one week, during which I hadn't noticed feeling anything other than my usual self, I came out of one particular meeting feeling tired, as though I could literally lie down and sleep. This was very unusual for me as I am not a daytime nap person at all - it has to be dark for me to sleep. I went for a coffee and sat in the staff room for a while, but couldn't shake off the tiredness. My manager came in and said that I looked washed out and when I explained how I was feeling, tired in my limbs, as though I could fall asleep, she insisted that I went straight to hospital because this was so unlike me. I just wanted to go home and sleep, but agreed that I would go to the hospital to get checked out.

The doctor at the local Accident & Emergency department examined me and said that I was suffering from exhaustion. I should go home and have a complete rest for a couple of days - no television, no reading, nothing - just rest. I went home and did what the doctor ordered. I stayed in bed for the whole weekend, but when Monday came I felt just the same. I felt lethargic and limp, my head felt thick and fuzzy and my eyelids wanted to stay closed. I telephoned work and stayed in bed, thinking I must have some kind of flu or something similar.

After a couple of days I went to see my GP. He signed me off work for two weeks saying I was exhausted and needed the rest. Over that time, I got into the routine of getting up in the morning at around 10:30 am, dragging my duvet downstairs and lying on the sofa all day, watching television. I would then go to bed at around 9 pm. I couldn't even get up and make myself anything to eat and lived on food that needed little or no preparation, like food replacement shakes, fruit and crisps.

My partner didn't understand how I felt at all. He was used to me being full of energy and life, wanting to go out and do things, not staying at home and dozing. He would go out to work in the morning leaving me in bed and come home in the evening to find me curled up on the sofa. He would look around and see that I had done no housework whilst I had been at home all day and he didn't understand why, when I wasn't really suffering from a *proper illness* – I was just tired! No one understood. Neither my Mum nor my friends could understand what had literally 'knocked me down' either and they visited trying to get me to go out, saying it would help to get me back to normal if I just 'made the effort'. People told me to "pull yourself together", that it was 'mind over matter', that just getting on with life would be enough to get me back to my normal self.

One of my neighbours, knowing that I love reading, brought me a pile of books. I began reading and this was what made me realise that there was something really wrong. I started a light novel and about ten pages in I came across the name Claire. "Who's Claire?" I thought, and flicked back to check. Claire was the character I had been reading about from the start and her name was on every page! I sat and cried. I thought I was going mad, that there must be something seriously wrong with me.

My GP referred me to a specialist, and after I had had every test imaginable, including a full MRI scan, he diagnosed me with M.E.

So, now I could go home and tell everyone that it was M.E. The only thing I remembered about ME. was 'Yuppy Flu', which was how it was reported when it had first emerged into the public consciousness. There was no internet, so I couldn't Google for information about it, and most importantly, I didn't know how I could get better – and I *so* wanted to get better. The doctors told me that there was no cure, and my GP asked if, when I got some information, I could tell him about it, because he knew nothing about it either!

Every day was a struggle. A struggle to muster the energy to go downstairs, a struggle to make lunch and a struggle to try to tidy up so that my partner would think that I had made an effort to do *something*.

After two months I found an organisation called Action for ME. They sent me leaflets about ME, which was most useful for the people around me and, of course, my GP.

I started taking magnesium supplements and Co-enzyme Q10. As the weather became warmer, I began to sit outside, enjoying the fresh air and the outdoors, which I had missed whilst staying inside.

After three months of a complete physical breakdown in terms of being able to function normally, I began to see some improvement in my symptoms. My partner took me to a local shopping centre and wheeled me around in a wheelchair so that I could get out a bit more and he would take me for drives in the countryside. I had particularly missed the countryside, as when I was well we used to go there every weekend to get out of the city suburbs where we lived.

I found that I would have very short periods of low energy, enabling me to get dressed or go round to my neighbour's house for a coffee. This energy would not last very long but it gave me hope that I was getting better. It was as though my batteries would charge up but run down very quickly, so I was limited in what I could do but I was seeing a glimmer of sunshine from behind the cloud.

The improvements continued very slowly but I gradually increased my level of physical activity. If I did too much I would know, because any period of over-activity would be followed by total incapacity again, so I was extremely careful to not push myself beyond what I felt able to do and as soon as I felt even slightly tired, I stopped and rested. After five months of gradual improvement I went to my employers to talk about returning to work part-time. Twelve months after I first became ill I returned to work full-time. I still had to pace myself and I had to become more efficient and more assertive.

Since my illness however, my outlook had changed. I now valued life outside of work more and I learned to say 'no' and be more disciplined in what I agreed to do and what I refused to take on – both at work and at home. I still enjoyed my job but I didn't work twelve hour days any more. I stopped being the ambitious and work-focused person I had been and reassessed my life. My life changed as I began to see work only as a way to earn money, and to enjoy a life outside work.

For several years following my illness I had 'good days' and 'bad days'. On 'good days' I felt 'normal' again, but if I overdid things, had a particularly late night or didn't listen to my body when it was saying '*stop*', I suffered for it with a bad day. Sometimes, I would think I had got away with it, but the bad day would always come, if not the next day then within a couple of days. On a typical bad day, I would struggle to get up in the morning, be tired and irritable all day and would have to rest.

Gradually, the 'good days' became more frequent and then it became rare for me to have a bad day. My partner and I split up and sold our house. I met my husband and moved away.

Now I am married with three young children – something I would never have imagined in the days before my illness. My life has turned out very differently to how it might have, had I never suffered from such a debilitating illness.

Two years after meeting my husband we had our first child. My experience of tiredness and ME stood me in good stead because, as every parent knows, the one thing that no parent-craft class can prepare you for is the sleep deprivation that a baby brings! I put into practice what I had done in the early days of recovery. I listened to my body and I slept when I needed to. Afternoon naps were back and I coped OK.

Seven months after our second child was born, I returned to university to study Environmental Biology. This was a three-year course that involved laboratory and field work and many long walks over steep, former spoil heaps. I did this, whilst working part time on Saturdays and Sundays and during my second year, whilst being pregnant with our third child, who was born on the day that I should have taken the first of my end of year exams. I then took my exams whilst nursing a four-week-old baby. I was delighted to complete my BSc with honours and achieved a 2:1. As I had enjoyed my studies so much, I decided that I wanted to continue. I was lucky enough to obtain a Research Studentship and I now spend time in muddy fields doing research towards my PhD.

Although it took time, a lot of patience and much perseverance, I can now do the things that I used to do in the days before M.E. My children, two boys now aged eight and three and a girl aged five, need me to be active and healthy. On reflection, getting my physical strength back seems easy, compared with regaining my mental strength. I lost so much confidence and the independent streak that had been so fierce before my illness had disappeared, making me constantly in need of company and feeling as though I could never cope alone. These were the other major impacts of ME, and it is probably these things which have taken the longest time to recover. Confidence needs re-building and self-assurance was something that I was sure I would never find again.

Thankfully I was wrong, I *can* cope; I could take the world on if I needed to and it has been my children who have proved this to me. Last year in March my husband had a lot of work to do, so I took all three children to Cumbria for a week to give him some peace and quiet. We had a great time, flying kites on the beach, digging sand and finding new places; we drove across the border and explored a Scottish castle and really enjoyed ourselves. It was very hard work and I salute single parents everywhere because there were a couple of times when I really could have done with the support of someone, so I could take time out to re-charge. But, the important thing is, that I did it. I managed. I coped. It was a revelation to me too, because even on the day that we were going, I had my doubts about whether anyone would last the week.

My three children love swimming and I swim with my daughter every week after her swimming lesson. We rarely have quiet 'family days' and when we are all together, we enjoy days out, most often somewhere that we can have 'adventures'. This usually involves a lot of walking through the countryside and finding forests that we can explore. The weather does not deter us and our motto is "the dirtier you are – the more fun you've had!" so muddy fields are fine for squelching through in our wellies!

I am very grateful that I have made an excellent recovery. I know that it is possible to recover, to regain my mental alertness and to be happy. In fact, when I was twenty-three, life *was* pretty good, but now I know that it is possible for it to be even better, because now I appreciate life so much more!

Most useful aid to recovery - positive thought and determination

Recommended website - www.afme.co.uk

Tracey's advice - I truly believe that positive thought and determination were the main things that helped me to recover. Recovery *is* possible and you *can* get a good quality of life again after ME. One thing you must do is *believe it!*

Tracey

Stuart's Story

The fog lifts

I am a thirty-eight year old male, now completely recovered from chronic fatigue syndrome/ME. As I think that my experiences may help others suffering with CFS, here is my story.

I have always been an active person, someone who worked hard and played hard, perhaps burning the candle at both ends a little too much. Going back a few years before I became ill, there were regular periods where I worked large amounts of overtime to meet deadlines, often working seventy-plus hours a week. I 'relaxed' by going down to the local pub for a few pints, although I never drank excessively. What free time I had was taken up with socialising or a number of different activities, including fencing at the local sports centre.

I met my wife in 1999 and got engaged in 2000, planning to marry in the summer of 2001. Gradually I found that I stopped going out so much and spent more time staying in. Work also calmed down to more of a steady routine, without the need for so much overtime.

In the autumn of 2000 organisational changes at work created a period of uncertainty and the pressure of work rose again over the following few months. Whereas previously I had enjoyed the challenge of my work and was happy with any pressure, this time the pressure was different and caused by, to a degree, poor management. I found myself having to do two jobs at once and was under increasing stress.

In February 2001 I became increasingly ill, initially trying to work through it but eventually admitting defeat and going to the doctor. I was told I had a particularly nasty throat infection and was placed on antibiotics and told to take ten days off work. After ten days I returned to work. Though the chaos I had left had somewhat abated and I wasn't so busy, I found myself struggling, still feeling awful and completely lacking in energy. I went back to my GP and after a series of blood tests showing I had suffered a major viral infection, my GP diagnosed post viral fatigue. He said I would feel tired for a few weeks but that I should be fine within a couple of months. I was told to take things easy and make sure I had plenty of fruit and vegetables in my diet. So, not unduly worried I just got on with things.

After 1st April the planned organisational changes at work left me with less work to do than I had been used to and I found this difficult, feeling very sleepy in the afternoons and struggling to work my full hours. I found myself increasingly using leave to take 'long weekends' but feeling just as tired the following Monday morning as I had at the end of the previous week.

By late May, I was getting concerned. I was no better and with the wedding set for August we were beginning to have to sort things out. I went back to my GP who said that he couldn't help me. I had further blood tests, which showed nothing, and my GP just suggested that I continue to take things easy.

I was much worse by the time August came. I had struggled on at work and had had a few more days off sick. I was hoping that a two week break in the sun on our honeymoon would prove to be the tonic that I needed.

I enjoyed my wedding day but wasn't able to enjoy it as much as I would have if I had been fit and healthy. I arrived in Mexico for the honeymoon feeling exhausted, but as the honeymoon was a once in a lifetime holiday I was determined to make the most of it; so we arranged for several all day excursions. I enjoyed them at the time, relaxing on the days in between, and by the end of the two weeks I wasn't feeling too bad. Although looking back now, it was clear that

I was storing up problems that would come back to haunt me in the near future.

I had a few days to rest when we got home before resuming work. Once back at work I was able to cope for only a couple of weeks before feeling appalling again. I went back to my GP and managed to get across that I was having real problems. She mentioned chronic fatigue syndrome and recommended that I take a month off work, but she wasn't able to offer any more advice than that. By this time, I was desperate so I agreed. I told work and then settled down at home for complete rest.

Within a week I was much, much worse. It was as though I had just kept going on adrenaline alone and now that had all gone I felt several times worse than the worst I had ever felt with flu. I became pretty much confined to the house. After a month I was no better and my GP wrote me off for another month.

About this time I started to research CFS/ME on the internet and came across a number of supplements that seemed to help a number of people. I had already tried high potency Aloe Vera, recommended by a relative, and that had had no effect, so now I tried Enzyme Co-Q10 which seemed to promise miracles. After a couple of weeks I seemed to have improved a little bit. I decided to take another month off work 'just to make sure' which would take me up to Christmas of 2001. I planned to return to work fully refreshed in January of 2002. However, just before Christmas, and seemingly for no reason, I went downhill rapidly. I became incredibly frustrated and more than a little depressed. My GP continued to say that there was nothing wrong with me and suggested that it may be psychological, rather than physical.

The next thing I tried was Enada NADH, which again seemed to promise miracles but was a little pricey, and by now after three months off work I was beginning to worry about the financial side of things. I was in a really bad way now. On good days I was able to move about the house without too much discomfort, but on the bad days, which seemed to be increasing in number, I was practically bedbound. This continued for over a month. During this time I experienced periods of deep depression and feelings of total inadequacy, some days not being too bad, other days feeling almost suicidal. I was also in almost constant pain.

My new wife was also finding things incredibly difficult. Although trying to be sympathetic and helpful she struggled to understand how the person she had met and fallen in love with had disappeared and her dreams of how enjoyable married life should be were shattered by the reality of having to care for a near total invalid. We both started having black moods and began to row, which further increased my feelings of despair and depression.

Very slowly I gradually improved again. By now I was also taking L-Carnitine in addition to the NADH and had also tried wearing magnetic bracelets and doing gentle yoga, both of which had been recommended to me. But I couldn't tell you whether anything was having any real benefit or not.

By March my sick pay had been exhausted and I was on benefits. Although my wife worked full time her wage was not enough to support both of us and I couldn't get anything more than the standard disability allowance, so I was keen to return to work as soon as possible. After discussions with both my GP and a work appointed GP, it was agreed that I attempt to return to work part time in April, doing just those hours I felt able to. Eager to be earning again, I started back at work on 4th April 2002.

By now I had finally joined Action for ME and noticed an advertisement for the 'Integrated Medical Practice' at Market Harborough, UK. At this point I was desperate and nothing that I had tried so far had made any real difference. I made an appointment. The drive to the clinic, though only forty miles, was the furthest I had driven in over a year, so was quite painful, but the consultation and the tests they undertook were not uncomfortable. The tests showed I that had a number of things wrong with me. It was a great relief that there were real physical problems that could be explained.

I had a picture taken of my blood that showed that my red blood cells were 'stuck' together in clumps, indicating poor digestion of protein. There was also evidence of a yeast infection in my blood and a sluggish lymphatic system. Other tests showed that my system was too acidic and that I was suffering from a variety of toxic heavy metal poisoning. All these indicated that I was suffering from a poor quality diet, a digestive system unable to absorb nutrients from that diet and a depressed immune system. I was told that these tests could certainly cause the poor health that I was experiencing and I was advised to change my diet and take a number of supplements. I was to cut down on sugar and processed foods and eat lots of fruit and vegetables with some supplements like high dose vitamin C and chlorella. An appointment was made for two months time to check on my progress.

I left feeling happy that finally something had been identified as wrong with me and that I could be treated, but angry that my GP couldn't offer me these kinds of tests on the National Health Service. Although I was still very cautious that this might prove to be another false hope and that nothing would improve, I felt that had I had these tests twelve months previously I may not have had to suffer the pain and depression that I had.

Initially the changes to my diet were a bit of an effort, but I soon got used to them. Within a month I was genuinely feeling better and the biggest change was that the constant heavy fog that I had seemed to be under all the time, had 'lifted'. Although I was still physically tired I was feeling mentally alert for the first time in over a year! This was something different. It seemed that, though at first nothing seemed to happen, gradually there was a real improvement, something tangible and noticeable, and my general mood really picked up.

By the time of the second set of tests eight weeks later, I had extended my hours at work and felt much, much better. The second set of tests showed that there had been some improvement but that there was still room for more, so I should continue with the diet and supplements.

By the summer I was able to take a near normal holiday for two weeks and actually enjoy it! I was also able to drive reasonably long distances. I still had to be careful, and several times over-did things, which resulted in my feeling tired for a while. But by December I was practically back at work full time!

A third set of tests showed that my blood was near normal. My red blood cells were no longer clumping together. There was no evidence of a yeast infection and it showed healthy white blood cells and a clear lymphatic system.

I resumed full-time work. I still got tired, but probably in the same way that anyone is tired after a days work. I still couldn't do everything I would like to and still had to be careful, but I was continuing to improve. I continued to take some supplements to maintain my health. The difference from ten months previously was huge. I found myself running upstairs whereas previously I had had to drag myself - and it had hurt.

It had been a long struggle. But the time period from February 2001 when I first suffered the virus which was the trigger, to the point where I felt near normal, was only two years. That's nothing compared to some people with ME. Had I had the tests at the Integrated Medicine Practice in February 2001, I believe that I could have been healthy again far more quickly.

I would thoroughly recommend anyone to check out the website and get in touch with the clinic to make an appointment. It is a private clinic so you do have to pay, but the few hundred pounds that I spent were spent willingly to avoid all the pain and misery. In an ideal world the NHS would offer these tests, but unfortunately they don't.

I could have made things easier for myself in other ways. I found myself having unrealistic expectations. I kept saying to myself, "I'll be better in a month" and was then disappointed when I wasn't, and I was disappointed when I tried one supplement or 'cure' only to have it not work. The good thing with the Integrated Medicine Practice is that each supplement recommended is targeted specifically at one or more of the problems that the tests show up, and in my case they worked relatively quickly. It took seven months from my first visit to the clinic to having almost normal test results and returning to full-time work.

I am fully aware and must emphasise that what worked for me may not work for everyone with ME. It is clear that rather than one cause, there is a whole raft of different things that cause the symptoms associated with ME, but it has to be common sense that one of the first things to do is to have detailed blood tests to see if there are any problems which may be causing the symptoms.

In my case, live blood analysis, the examination of a blood sample immediately after drawing it, showed up a number of things that NHS blood tests wouldn't even look for. Then bio-terrain analysis, something considered on the fringes of 'proper' medicine, confirmed a number of additional problems linked to poor nutrition. All of these problems could be addressed relatively simply with a change of diet, or specific supplements and clearing up these problems also cleared up my symptoms.

Now, some six years after my initial illness, I am continuing to work full time without problems. I am still somewhat unfit and not perhaps as generally healthy as I was previously, but I am probably no worse than the majority of the population and would consider myself fully 'cured'. My work involves foreign travel and long haul flights - no problem; long hours at work - no problem. The odd missed nights sleep, I can take in my stride. General illness no longer holds the fears that it did a few years ago. I have suffered from a couple of nasty viral illnesses over the last year or so, and come through them with no long term ill-effects.

I can fully appreciate and enjoy life again. There isn't much that I can't do. I won't be running in the Olympics any time soon (!) but I can manage and enjoy just about everything I did beforehand. We have wonderful long days out, like going to the zoo which involves a lot of walking, and I can drive long distances again without problems. In short, apart from a lower level of overall fitness, which I keep intending to do something about, I suffer no long term ill effects from my experience. There were effects other than physical though; my marriage nearly didn't survive and we had to work hard through a long bad patch in order to save it. ME effects a lot more than just the individual's health and it can be just as hard and frustrating for loved ones and friends, something not always recognised. But we are happy now and perhaps appreciate life a little more than we did.

Most useful aid to recovery - Integrated Medical Practice

Recommended websites
www.bioterrain.co.uk
www.liveblood.co.uk
www.positivehealthshop.com

Stuart's advice - don't give up, but don't have unrealistic expectations, take things slowly and steadily. Appreciate life as fully as you are able. I had someone put a bird feeder in my back garden and just sitting and watching the birds gave me a lot of pleasure when I was low. And above all, remember that there is always someone worse off than yourself.

Stuart Runham

Lilla's story

It's going to be a bright, bright sun-shiny day

Having managed my energy and life for six years after severe ME, which initially lasted about two years, it returned with force. I didn't know how I'd got well the first time; whether it was the touch for health healing, the acupuncture, the wheat free diet, the healing symbol therapy, the meditation, the supplements, the journalling, my will - or a raft of other approaches I'd tried.

That familiar helpless feeling was back. I had no energy to exercise, socialise, or work. It was like trying to look down a blind alley with a bag over my head and my hands tied behind my back. I spent months in a fog valiantly researching the Internet for some insight into the cause of ME and importantly *anything* I could do that would effect permanent change and put my life back in my own hands.

When I came across Phil Parker's training, through a friend who had heard of him on the radio, I wasn't at all sure this would work for *me*. My natural intelligence and intuition was out of whack and when I asked myself the question 'do you want to be well and healed of M.E.?' back came the answer 'No, I don't want to leave the house, or go into the world and make a living, or stop receiving all this loving support from friends, or take responsibility for myself'. Recognising it was important to include these responses, I then moved through them in moments to a resounding 'Yes, I *do* want to be well'.

From that moment on I was committed to my journey and the training and ready to get all the value I could stand. I was really willing to put the work in. Money flowed to me, including winning one hundred pounds on the Grand National and I started to reconnect with the heart of being back in the driving seat of my life.

From the second day of applying The Lightning Process training with gusto and determination, I was awake at 7am, happy, walking for a mile or two, clear headed and present in the world.

A week later I taught two classes of children and felt energised! I walked for an hour or more a day, gardened, worked on my book and a design commission, partied, and started going to bed at midnight. I found myself singing out loud that song, 'I can see clearly now the rain is gone, I can see all obstacles in my way, gone are the dark clouds that had me blind, it's going to be a bright, bright sun-shiny day' ......
which is close to a metaphor for the Lightning Training for me.

Most useful aid to recovery - The Lightning Process

Recommended website - www.lightningprocess.com

Lilla

Alexandra's Story

I had to change the *balance* of my diet

I first became ill in 1985 when I was twenty-six years old. I was working as a radio production assistant during the week and moonlighting as a staff nurse at weekends. Like so many people I caught flu and 'never recovered'. I was diagnosed with ME within a few months but went on to be ill for the next four years. I staggered into work when I could and was off work sick, often for months at a time, when I couldn't.

I was a nurse, yet I had never heard of an illness like ME. I had a lot of upsetting visits with disbelieving doctors who thought I was just depressed because, despite my diagnosis, they had never heard of ME either. One day I heard about a doctor who believed that ME was a physical condition and I went to see him privately. He organised blood tests which showed that I was deficient in various vitamins and minerals, particularly magnesium, and told me that I suffered from 'rocky blood sugar levels'. He advised me to 'eat protein and carbohydrates together regularly' and take vitamin and mineral supplements. Having been more or less bed-bound at the stage I saw him and needing a wheelchair to go out, I have photographs of me six months later running around the zoo with my one-year-old son on my shoulders.

I felt fit, healthy and happy then for about seven years. I worked part-time at the BBC whilst my son was at school. I did aerobics and dance classes, went skiing on holiday and had no symptoms of ME at all during this time.

Three or four years in, however, not understanding how important my diet was, I stopped being careful about eating regular protein and stopped taking supplements. I returned to what is widely advised as a 'healthy' low fat diet. Although I was very happy with my life, I noticed a return of the emotional dips which I had had since I was a child, when I would feel sad for 'no reason'. I found I was either feeling low, or I was eating regular sugar and caffeine to 'give me a lift'. I never put the two together. I always thought I was feeling down because of something else going on in my life. Later I began to wake up in the night feeling sad, angry or just wakeful, only able to feel fine again and return to sleep after a large bowl of cereal! I had no idea I was self-medicating low blood sugar levels.

In the few years before I got ill the second time, I increased my work hours, remarried, moved house twice and had another baby. Immediately afterwards we moved into a cramped one-room basement flat for several months whilst our new house was turned into a building site and treated with dry rot chemicals. When we returned to a house full of builders I went to the doctor saying that I felt anxious and down. He diagnosed me with post-natal depression and gave me prozac. Being on prozac was like being on speed. For six months I barely ate, lived on coffee and couldn't sleep for more than five or six hours a night, but was consistently cheerful! I turned into what I thought was 'super-mum'. I went into a frenzy of cleaning and cooking and redecorating the newly repaired house. I went to dance classes two evenings a week and socialised and looked after my seven year old son and baby, often on my own as my husband was working abroad for several weeks at a time.

Six months after starting prozac I crashed. I woke up one day unable to get out of bed at all. The ME was back – wham – with little warning other than being a bit tired getting up in the mornings for a few months before. At first we kept our hopes up – it would be a three week relapse; a three month relapse; six months or even a year - but it ended up being another seven long years. And this time was more devastating than the last time, because I was worse than I was before and I had two children to look after.

I became an invalid. I was house-bound and often bed-bound. I couldn't look after my children or the house, let alone myself, so we had to get a live-in, full-time au-pair for five years, and my husband operated as a single father evenings and weekends. I remember feeling devastated when my toddler thought that a mummy duck with her ducklings in a picture book was a daddy duck. I couldn't make a shopping list, understand what people were saying to me or remember how to finish a sentence. I slept nineteen out of twenty-four hours for several years. I slept right through my son's ninth birthday and prised my eyes open only long enough to watch him blow the candles out. Just walking the length of the kitchen felt like climbing Mount Everest with a ten ton elephant on my back. Needless to say, I got very depressed. Eventually I used a wheelchair or disabled scooter for the rare family outing.

My doctor took a blood test showing flattened red blood cells which he said looked like malnutrition "but can't possibly be because you're in England and not Africa". He also took a test showing high prolactin levels, because I was still producing milk four years after stopping feeding my baby. All other tests came back normal. He gave me low-dose amitriptyline for the night-time insomnia and continuous, all-over muscle pain and I took it for four years. In the first year of taking it I put on three stone, so I spent the next five years in leggings and T-shirts because I was too ill to go shopping – at least they were ideal for in bed and out. When I came off the amitriptyline I realised it had turned me into even more of a zombie than I already was and had also given me some of the strange side-effects that had worried me so much over the years.

The NHS were unable to help further so like many people I tried lots of different alternative therapies – some of which were very helpful. I tried osteopathy, Chinese medicine, homeopathy, reiki, spiritual healing, reflexology, counselling, various diets, hypnotherapy, yoga – you name it, I tried it – right down to colonic irrigation.

Later I went to private doctors and had tests done showing gut dysbiosis, reactive hypoglycaemia, low adrenal (cortisol) output, low thyroid levels, raised oestrogen, vitamin and mineral deficiencies, blood abnormalities like the misshapen red blood cells and clotting and so on. I was given adrenal and thyroid hormones for a year or so according to Dr Jacob Teitelbaum's protocol and I felt better on them.

As my brain began to come back I started researching. ME is, after all, only a collection of symptoms and I was determined to find out what was causing them, because something certainly was. I was desperate to get well for my children. I was saddened by the effect my illness was having on them and I was determined that I would recover in time to be a good mum to them. Getting well became my full-time job and every day I tried to do everything right – eat the right food, take the right supplements, do the right exercise, rest, meditate, walk so many steps … and so on. I was constantly starting new protocols and regimes. As each one failed, I tried another. But everything I tried helped me. Everything took me another step forward - if only because every book I read, every new supplement, exercise or routine I tried, gave me the hope I needed to keep going.

I spent much of my time studying on the Internet and reading the many books I bought from Amazon on health, nutrition, spirituality, mind/body medicine, psychology and personal development. I was particularly interested in studying the commonalities between people who recovered from 'incurable' illnesses. Although as a nurse I was sceptical of the idea that diet had much to do with health, it was diet that came up time and time again. Diet and/or peace of mind appeared to be the two keys to recovery. So I decided to address both.

I learned about mind/body medicine and the power of the mind and I put as much as possible into practice, including meditation, relaxation, self-hypnosis and positive thinking. Autogenics I found particularly helpful. I learned that my mind and body were one and the same, and that the health of each were dependent upon the other.

I learned that a healthy body meant a naturally positive mind, and vice versa. I learned that stressful thoughts produce stressful hormones which are not conducive to healing, so I learned how to change what I was thinking about. I particularly liked a phrase of Anthony Robbin's "if you think what you have always thought, you will get what you have always got", demonstrating that I had to start changing the way I thought in order to get out of the mess I was in. Even if it only meant I had to stop thinking that I was helpless, and start thinking of a way out!

I became very interested in nutrition. I came across articles and books by doctors and nutritional scientists who believe that our modern, recommended 'low fat, high carbohydrate diet' has a tendency to cause unstable blood sugar levels and hormonal imbalance, and has contributed to the huge increase in chronic degenerative diseases like cancer, heart disease, diabetes and obesity and, possibly even, the recent 'epidemic' of CFS/ME – and it all made sense to me. I had tried different diets, including of course the anti-candida diet; I had taken lots of supplements and cut out sugar, wheat and dairy products, but I had continued to eat a low fat diet based around carbohydrates, eating rice cakes by the ton load. Regular carbohydrates, I had found, were the only thing that made me feel even *half*-human, but now I realised I didn't need all those carbohydrates to keep my blood sugar levels stable, and that it was, in fact, all those carbohydrates which were *causing* the problem. I had *far too many* carbohydrates in my diet and not enough fat or protein to balance the resultant rocky blood sugar levels. I finally understood that it was the *balance* of my diet which was wrong.

I learned that when you eat something sweet or refined it causes a rapid increase in blood sugar levels and then a massive drop below normal. The brain can't function without glucose for more than a few minutes so it sends very powerful biochemical messages urging you to eat something sweet quickly. You feel this as a 'need' to eat or even a craving. It is very difficult to ignore these survival messages from the brain, because if you do, you suffer the effects of low blood sugar, a result of a brain deprived of glucose. Many people suffer low blood sugar levels all their lives without realising it, self-medicating with a cup of coffee and a biscuit, afternoon tea, a bed-time snack to 'give them a lift'. Many others like me, try to avoid these foods for their health or to avoid weight gain and are made fully aware of the powerful effect of low blood sugar levels. Low blood sugar levels can make us feel depressed, tired, irritable, anxious, foggy brained, forgetful, light-headed, confused, weak, craving sweet foods, hungry and wakeful at night. Chronically low blood sugar levels can make us feel like that all the time – and we unconsciously try to improve the situation by continually eating sugar, caffeine and anything else to give us a 'lift'.

My whole life suddenly made sense. My struggles with sugar, caffeine, nicotine at one time and even shift-work when nursing. My emotional dips, *solved* by any of the above stimulants. All these things were a cause, and a result, of rocky blood sugar levels. What I had thought was a 'normal' diet of cereal for breakfast, bread for lunch and pasta for tea, was actually a diet based around refined carbohydrates which was causing me blood sugar swings throughout the day and triggering a desire to eat sweet foods often. What had felt like an 'addiction' to sweet foods was simply a result of low blood sugar levels.

I learned that every time our blood sugar level drops our adrenal glands are triggered to pour out adrenaline in an attempt to balance them. This is the well-known 'fight or flight' response. Our adrenals were designed to cope with the occasional stressful situation of "oops, panic, there's a mammoth in our path". They were not designed to be continually triggered throughout the day, day after day and year after year, to raise chronically low blood sugar levels, caused by a diet high in sugar, refined carbohydrates and stimulants like caffeine. If the adrenals are over-worked then it seems that our stress hormones can become depleted and our ability to cope with stress, whether emotional or physical, is reduced. A low fat diet aggravates the situation because the adrenals need natural fats in order to make more stress hormones and if you aren't eating enough you can't make more.

I learned that rocky blood sugar levels and fatigued adrenal glands can cause hormonal havoc by unbalancing hormones like insulin, adrenaline, cortisol, thyroxine, growth hormone, oestrogen and progesterone and by depleting brain chemicals like serotonin (happiness) and dopamine (motivation). They can also depress the immune system, over-stimulate the central nervous system, disrupt digestion, keep the cardiac system on red alert and so on.

Having learned the connection between carbohydrates, blood sugar balance and the adrenal glands, I realised that the fashionable low fat, high carbohydrate diet which we have been told is 'healthy' over the last forty years and which I had been eating my entire life, might actually be *causing* my problems rather than alleviating them. So, five years after becoming ill, I decided to try a low carbohydrate diet. I was convinced that I would feel terrible without my normal intake of carbohydrates, and indeed I did, but only for the first five days.

The breakthrough came on day six when I woke up with a clear head in time to see the children off to school for the first time in five years! Usually it was a struggle to wake up before midday. And my brain fog had lifted! I even felt mildly cheerful! From then on I didn't look back. I cut out *man-made* carbohydrates, binned the rice cakes and continued eating essentially as our distant ancestors did - meat, fish, eggs, dairy, nuts, seeds, fruit and vegetables - and gradually my strength came back. At six months I no longer needed our live-in au-pair and at eighteen months I went canoeing in France on an active family camping holiday.

By changing to a low carbohydrate diet I had reduced the level of glucose in my blood and my blood sugar levels had stabilised. This meant that my adrenals were no longer being triggered throughout the day so they were able to recuperate, recover and replenish their supply of hormones. Adrenal stress tests showed my adrenal hormone levels gradually returning to within normal range, and as this happened, all my symptoms started disappearing, indicating that perhaps other systems were also returning to normal.

As well as reducing carbohydrates I increased protein and natural fats in my diet. I learned that every cell in our body is made out of protein and fat, from our brain chemicals to our organs to our muscles, and that we need enough protein and fat in order to be able to rebuild cells and produce hormones and repair daily damage – *especially* when we are sick. Nowadays we often don't eat enough protein and natural fats because we are filling up on too many man-made carbohydrates, which provide mainly glucose for energy. This is obviously fine if you are an athlete and can use up lots of them, but if you are an office worker you need less and if you are crashed out with ME, like I was, then you really don't need many at all. Bearing in mind that the only form of carbohydrates our distant ancestors ate were fruit and vegetables and that farming cereal grains began only 10,000 years ago, a 'blink of an eye' in genetic terms, then you can see how some of us may not yet have adapted very well to toast for breakfast, sandwiches for lunch and pasta for tea. Especially considering the huge increase in *refined* grains in our diet over the last fifty years.

I had dismissed gluten intolerance as being a contributory factor of my illness because as a nurse I had learned that coeliac disease presented with bowel problems, which I hadn't had; and I had already cut out wheat, a major source of gluten, within a few years of getting ill. However, after I recovered from ME I learned that gluten intolerance/ coeliac disease can present without bowel problems and can be an underlying cause of fatigue, depression and nutrient deficiencies, as well as blood sugar and hormonal problems. So I got myself tested. My blood tests indicated severe gluten intolerance and a high likelihood of coeliac disease. In order to get a definite diagnosis here in the UK you have to go back on gluten for two months and undergo an endoscopy. Having eaten very little gluten for four years I was pleased to have the opportunity of eating bread and pasta again to my hearts delight, however, my doctor and I abandoned that route after one month back on gluten left me depressed, unable to wake up in the morning, ten pounds over-weight and with horrible stomach and bowel problems. I didn't need to suffer another month for an endoscopy to tell me that gluten was a problem for me after all. One doctor I saw suggested that my gluten intolerance may have been the entire underlying cause of my ME. He said that untreated gluten intolerance can cause blood sugar problems and eventual low adrenal and thyroid function, which seemed to fit in with my tests and symptoms.

Six months after my change in diet my stool tests returned showing that I no longer had the klebsiella and candida infections that I had been battling for five years and I was no longer mal-absorbing proteins and fats. My red blood cells looked fine and my adrenal hormone levels returned to within normal range within the year, as did my vitamin B12 and magnesium levels. My blood pressure no longer dropped on standing and my skin rash disappeared. I did however still have reactive hypoglycaemia, which obviously I suffered from even as a child, and which is so common today. This means that if I eat sugar or refined carbohydrates, my blood sugar levels swing hugely upwards and then crash very low, leaving me feeling emotional, irritable and tired – and craving more sugar or caffeine to raise them again quickly.

As I was recovering, I began to feel 'normal' doing nothing. At this stage I began to work on building up my strength. I started walking five minutes to the end of the road and kept this going for a week. I then increased it to ten minutes for another week, and so on. It was a long, slow process, but after about six months I was walking for half-an-hour twice a day and after that I didn't even need to think about it.

As I got physically better I initially became more anxious. Probably because the big wide world was coming back for me to deal with and when you've been cocooned in your home for so many years it all seems a bit much. I also struggled with depression. I needed to 'move on', but I was stuck grieving the loss of so many years of a normal family life with the children. I was also learning to manage my blood sugar levels. Also, according to the Coeliac Association, it can take a year of *strict* adherence to a gluten free diet for serotonin (happiness) and dopamine (motivation) metabolite concentrations in the brain to increase again to normal levels. So all in all, my physical health returned first and my brain dragged along behind! There was also a lot of readjusting to do for my husband and me. We had to relearn how to deal with each other as partners rather than invalid and carer. It wasn't easy. After so many years of being strong and holding everything together, he was exhausted too.

So what do I think was wrong with me? Of course I don't know for sure, but given that I recovered both times by balancing my blood sugar levels, I *suspect* that my poor health was the end-result of my susceptibility to the high amount of sugar and gluten in our highly refined western diet. I *suspect* that I had, as a result, 'less-than-buoyant' adrenal glands, which were only able to cope as long as everything went along relatively easily in my life, and when I had one stress too many, as I did twice, then they could not cope and down I went with ME.

And if gluten, rocky blood sugar levels and the hormonal consequences weren't the entire cause of my ME, then they must surely have played a part in making me susceptible to whatever does cause it, perhaps due to a consequently depleted immune system.

As our adrenal glands are triggered by both emotional and physical stress, I believe that I could also have recovered if I had been able to reduce my emotional stress, which I certainly had my share of. However, I think that without changing my diet as well, my recovery would have been forever dependent on maintaining a stress-free life, because as long as my adrenals were being continually triggered by a less than optimal diet, they were never going to regain full strength. As it was, changing my diet meant that my adrenals became strong enough to cope with the emotional stresses that I had, as they were designed to do.

So how did I recover from ME? The answer for me was simple in the end. I changed the *balance* of the diet I had eaten for most of my life. I changed from a low fat, high carbohydrate diet which we have all been told since the 1970s is good for our health – to a lower carbohydrate diet with increased protein and natural fats which balanced my blood sugar levels, restored my hormonal balance, strengthened my immune system and provided the raw materials to rebuild and repair my body and brain.

I hope that if I remain gluten-free and maintain balanced blood sugar levels (as our ancestors naturally did) that my adrenal glands will protect me well enough from the effects of stress for the rest of my life and allow the rest of my body to work as it should. I believe that by maintaining my changed diet *and* dealing promptly with my emotional stresses, that I have the best chance of a sustained recovery and good health in the future.

Now, as long as I am careful to keep *man-made* carbohydrate levels low, then I can cope cheerfully with anything that life throws at me. But, if I succumb to sugary temptation and keep it up for a few days, then I will experience fluctuating blood sugar levels with depression as a result; and I will find it harder to wake up in the morning. It takes five days off sugary foods for me to feel good again. I owe it to my family to be vigilant about my diet so that it never again leads to what I suspect was the end-result – ME.

It took me a long time to unravel what was wrong with me, and then to correct it. I hope very much that it doesn't take you as long to find out what is causing your own illness, and I wish you all the very best for a return to your own good health.

Most useful aid to recovery - a strong reason to get well (my children). A fierce determination to get back to full health whatever the cost and do whatever it took. A refusal to believe anyone who said it wasn't possible.

Recommended books
"Life Without Bread – How a Low Carbohydrate Diet Can Save Your Life" by Dr Wolfgang Lutz**
"Nourishing Traditions – The Cookbook that Challenges Politically Correct Nutrition and the Diet Dictocrats" by Sally Fallon &

Mary G Enig, Ph.D
"Protein Power" by Dr Eades
"Tired of Being Tired – Do you Have Adrenal Burnout?" by Dr Jesse Lynn Hanley
"From Fatigued to Fantastic" by Dr Jacob Teitelbaum
"Be Your Own Life Coach" by Fiona Harrold
"Molecules of Emotion – Why You Feel The Way You Feel" by Candace B Pert, Ph.D
"Being Happy" by Andrew Matthews
"The Magic of Thinking Big" by David Schwartz

Recommended websites
www.westonaprice.org
www.fionaharrold.com
www.coeliac.co.uk
www.endfatigue.com
www.dymyhill.co.uk

Alexandra's advice –Removing stress can help the body to heal so it can be helpful to make a simple list of all your physical and your emotional stresses and then start dealing with them, one at a time, starting with the easiest.

Quote - "Never, never, never, never give up". Winston Churchill

Alexandra Barton

Joy's Story

Two hours after the first dose I felt
the ME symptoms roll away

I had ME for eight and a half years and was diagnosed by four doctors and two professors. I was seventy-one and felt that I would be too old to appreciate it if I ever did get better, but in the summer of 2002 I consulted a professor in London. After a few false starts he suggested that I had a urine test for thyroid function, which, at the time, was only done in Holland. The results showed very low readings for T3 and T4. The National Health Service had never shown anything other than normal levels for T4 and had never tested for T3. I didn't present as a thyroid case either, which can be attested to by my present GP and the professor.

My readings were: T3   184 : mean ref. value in urine   1400-2500
                   T4   309 : mean ref. value in urine   1800-3000

I was prescribed Thyroxine and Tertroxin and, here is the amazing part, two hours after the first dose I felt all the ME symptoms roll away! That was at the end of October 2002 - and I am still feeling perfectly normal six years later.

I had to get my strength back, of course, as I used to use an electric buggy to get about. However, before long I could stride about with no

exhaustion and no blank head. The relief was extraordinar
my life back!

I want to let the world know that this thyroid test is som..
worth trying. I'm sure I can't be the only person to have had 'normal'
thyroid tests done on the NHS when they are not normal at all. T3 isn't
usually tested in the NHS blood test as it is thought to be unnecessary
if the T4 level is normal. However, as T4 has to convert to T3, there
can be reasons why it's not converting.

Sometimes you need to treat the adrenals as well as the thyroid
to regain your health. Both work so closely together. If you are not
feeling good on thyroid hormone alone it could be worth having an
adrenal stress test to see whether you are producing enough adrenal
hormones. If you are not, then you can take adrenal supplements. By
having regular thyroid and adrenal tests, you can make sure that you
are taking the correct hormones/supplements and feeling as well as
possible.

Good luck to all of you, it is well worth a try! I was diagnosed with
ME, yet I was cured by thyroid hormone. I now keep an eye on both
my thyroid and adrenals and supplement when necessary. Do please
let me know if you follow this up and *do* believe me!

Most useful aid to recovery - Thyroid hormones

Recommended book - "The Great Thyroid Scandal" by Dr Barry
Peatfield

Recommended websites
www.thyroiduk.org
www.nptech.co.uk (for adrenal stress tests)
www.iwdl.net

Joy Anthony

Ri's Story

The Power of Forgiveness

If you have chronic fatigue syndrome, fibromyalgia or ME, then please listen up. The following message is for you if you are truly serious about healing yourself. You see, there is no doubt or question that you can heal. Your body is programmed for perfect health and has a Divine system to restore any imbalance or dis-ease. The question really isn't can you heal, the question that I have for you is...do you really want to heal? Now that may sound like a weird question to ask someone who is chronically sick. Bear with me please. What I am about to reveal can be a spring-board to your complete healing, that is if you are ready to hear the message.

I was chronically sick for over four years with a condition sometimes referred to as chronic fatigue syndrome. So, I can honestly say that I know from personal experience what it is like to be very sick for a long time period. If you are chronically sick with an autoimmune disease or any other type of health condition, then you know what it is like to feel terrible and have no one who can explain to you why. I went to numerous doctors and had many blood tests run over the span of three years. Nothing could explain why I felt so terrible.

I was very confused and scared to say the least. How could it be that a health conscious young man could feel so horrible and have all the passion that I once had, simply disappear from my life? How could

I wake up one morning and have my whole life change? Well, little did I know at that time what a long and bumpy road lay ahead of me.

You see there was an irony in my illness. I was an individual who was into health and taking care of my body as far back as high school. I worked out four to five days a week and ate typically very well. So, how was it that I got so sick that I could no longer participate in life like a normal person? I could no longer work out because I didn't have the energy or strength. I had to quit my job because I simply could no longer fulfill my duties as I once did. I no longer went out with my friends because I felt so horrible all the time and I did not have the will to do so. I couldn't even enjoy just sitting there because my condition took all enjoyment in my life away from me. The only peace I ever had was when I was asleep.

This may sound very familiar to you. So, what was going on with me? Did my illness just spring into being from nothingness? How could I become sick when I followed many health regimens to ensure that I didn't get sick in the first place? Well, knowing what I know now, it was a definite and sure sign that something was trying to get my attention.

After being sick for over three years without any explanation I had reached a point of complete exhaustion and depression. In fact, I didn't want to be on this planet any longer. All my dreams and goals seemed to be flushed down the toilet. I had no passion and wanted out of this game called life. As I sat there one day in my room, I was ready to give up on life. I was going to ask the universe to take me out and away from this misery. All of a sudden, it was as if the Universe hit me on the head with a sledge hammer. The message I received was profound. This all happened in a flash. In that one instant, I had an epiphany that would change my life forever. I finally realized that I had a choice. I could continue to sit there and feel sorry for myself and play the victim or I could take a stand to empower myself and restore my health. In that moment, I stood up and made a vow that I would heal myself and feel better than I ever had in my entire life. That day I realized that the universe is waiting for you to wake up and assume your power. The universe only responds to you when you vow to change your life. If you pray and feel hopeless and afraid, then the universe will not respond to you. Essentially, your vibration is the key to receiving help from the Infinite Spirit that created you. If you are in victim mode, then you will get no response. Show the universe that you are serious and watch what happens.

So, I made a total commitment to myself that I would unravel this mystery of chronic illness. I totally gave up on traditional doctors because they were more baffled and clueless than I was about my illness. As I learned through my personal experience, western medicine is only concerned about treating symptoms and not finding the true cause of illness. So I set out on a journey to find the true cause of my mystery illness. I spent endless hours researching every aspect of health and disease. The more I learned, the more I realized that holistic modalities are more effective in treating chronic illnesses. Holistic health modalities incorporate natural regimens to restore the body back to complete balance.

For many years I concentrated only on the physical level because that was what I was conditioned to believe in. Ever since I was a child and up until my illness, I had accepted the belief that illness is a physical manifestation and thus the cause must be physical as well. Boy, did I have a lot to learn! As I learned through my personal experience, most diseases do not primarily stem from a physical root cause. Environment and a person's diet can contribute to disease, however most diseases have deeper underlying root causes. If disease had strictly physical root causes then we would have a cure for almost every single illness on the planet.

As I continued to acquire more knowledge through my personal experience and through my research, I started to try some of the holistic therapies that I thought would help my condition. I used herbs, homeopathic remedies, chiropractic care, acupuncture, natural supplements, and energy therapies. I totally changed my diet to organic foods and even switched all my personal care products such as shampoo, soap, and toothpaste to all natural varieties. I had come so far and changed so much in my life. I did see improvements in my health after receiving some of these holistic therapies. However, why was it that after all these changes in my life and using natural therapies, I still did not feel completely well?

The answer was that I did not have a balance in my life of mind, body, and spirit! I was always so concerned about the physical aspects of my being that I neglected the most important parts of myself. I worked out and always made sure that I was well groomed and well dressed but I never gave even a thought to my mental, emotional and spiritual health. So, I started to expand my mind and learn many things about the mind, body, and spirit connection. I read many books on the topic and discovered some very profound information that seemed to light a fire inside of me. Everything that I discovered fit so perfectly, as to how and why I got sick and how to get myself back to complete health. It was amazing how dramatically my health was improving as I continued to incorporate more love and attention to my mind and my spirit and heal old emotional wounds. I had finally found the magic key to unlock the mystery of my illness. It all made such perfect sense now about the mystery of my illness and why I was sick for so long. The answers that I so desperately sought were within me the whole time! Similarly, the root cause to my illness began within me as well. However, now I had true understanding as to what happened and how I could fix it. I cannot even come close to explaining how happy and exhilarated I was to have my health improving as I continued to work on my mental and spiritual health. Of course I continued with taking care of myself physically, but I just didn't have to expend as much time and energy as I used to. It seemed almost as if the physical part of me was improving automatically as I worked to bring my emotions, my mind and spirit back into balance. It was amazing to see that by releasing old emotions and learning how to really forgive, that my physical health could take such quantum leaps in improvement!

So, here I sit today feeling better than I have ever felt in my life. I have a totally new outlook on life and have such high passion for everything I do. Having gone through my experiences with my illness, it has inspired me to finding my true purpose in life. I am a holistic health coach and have a passion for helping people to restore their health. I had the best education that I could ever find anywhere. My personal experiences have given me such profound knowledge about health and healing. I consider my past experiences with my illness a blessing in disguise because so much good has come from it. I feel better than I have ever felt and have a closer connection to my inner self. I have discovered all the knowledge that I need to help keep myself healthy. I have also found my true passion in life. I am now able to empower people to help themselves look and feel great. As I learned on my quest to heal myself, the biggest challenges in your life bring with them the biggest rewards.

You see, all illness, I don't care what you label it or what your doctor wants to label it, is a major sign from your spirit that you have made an error in the way you think and feel. What does this mean? It means that on some level of your being you have used your thoughts and emotions in a destructive way toward yourself and others.

Here are some facts for you. The following is not theory or philosophy. It is scientific fact and has been known by some for many years. More than 95% of all chronic illness is caused by internal stress (toxic emotions) created by your mind. Your emotions are the fuel for illness to manifest. Your emotions are the biggest killer of your immune system bar none. Your emotions suppress your immune system which in turn allows invaders such as viruses, parasites, candida (yeast) and other pathogens to take a firm hold on your body. Once they do, they sabotage most if not all of your organ systems and biochemical processes. They do this by dumping their wastes in your body and wreaking havoc on your major organs.

These invaders are not the cause of your illness. So called mystery viruses are also not the root cause for your illness. Your thyroid not working properly is not the cause of your illness. All the stuff you read about on the Internet is not the cause of your illness. Want to know the root cause of your illness right now? Are you sure? I help 95% of my clients get to the root cause of their illness in five minutes or less by asking one simple question. How do I do this? Simple, I use the wisdom I gained in going through my own experience.

I ask...who is the problem? You see something happened to you either right before you became ill or a number of months prior. I really don't care what happened but something occurred that caused you to have feelings of resentment, anger, hatred, and bitterness toward someone. It usually is a person. This is why I ask *who* is the problem. You will be surprised at what you discover if you can simply be honest with yourself. Someone broke your heart, someone fired you, someone cheated on you, someone made you feel small, someone deceived you, someone abandoned you, someone took away your child, someone stole from you, someone manipulated you, someone abused you and the list goes on and on. Whatever happened caused you severe emotional and mental stress for a long time period.

This shuts down your immune system and creates blockages in your energy fields. This means that your energy does not flow properly throughout your body. You are mainly an energetic being. Your health is dependent upon energy running smoothly throughout your organs and cells. When you become blocked energetically speaking, this energy cannot enter your cells for proper communication.

It is your stored emotions from the event that caused you grief and the energy blockages that are keeping you sick. I don't care what you do physically for your illness...it will not heal you. You must remove or transmute the emotions and energy blockages to restore your health. How do you do that? There is only one way to heal your illness. There is only one remedy for complete recovery. In fact, it is the one key to heal all life situations for every person alive today. It is called forgiveness. Forgive whoever hurt you, cheated on you, lied to you, fired you, abandoned you, abused you, yelled at you, demeaned you, and whatever else someone did to you.

Forgiveness is the most powerful healing force in the entire Universe. I guess Jesus knew this secret thousands of years ago. Boy was he ever right! When you really forgive someone, there are biochemical changes in your body immediately. The energy blockages all restore themselves.

Again, science has proven this as well. This is not new to some who have known this truth. My friend, it is time to let go and forgive. It doesn't matter what anyone did or said. Everyone makes mistakes and says and does things that hurt others. Keep in mind that some of these events may have happened in your childhood. You may be carrying a huge load from your childhood and are now feeling the effect. Look at your life and it will reveal the truth to you.

It all boils down to love. There are many life stories but really only one lesson. It is called *Love*. Somewhere deep down inside, you don't feel loved, supported, nurtured, appreciated or honored. You may have low self-esteem and self worth. It still boils down to Love. My friend, you must learn to love yourself and love life. You are perfect as you are. There is no need to become greater. All you have to do is let your true light shine. This is why you are here on this planet. You are here to gift the world with who you are. That is the secret to life. To just be who you are and love yourself and honour what you have to give the world.

My friend, it is time to heal. You simply must. If you choose to hold on for dear life you will perish and never allow your light to shine. This planet needs all the light it can have right now. If your light goes out, then there is less light for others to see with. It is your duty to heal. Just as you used your mind to plant seeds of illness, you can now shift and use it to plant new seeds, ones of health, vitality, happiness and peace. You choose!

If you really want to heal, then it's time to deal! To Your Health!

Most useful aid to recovery - forgiveness

Recommended book - any books by Carolyne Myss are wonderful.

Useful quote - "Make Your Destiny, Don't Let Destiny Make You!"

Ri

Lizzie's story

A frank ode to my life-altering friend and nemesis

An all consuming, debilitating, dream-crushing illness is what really lies behind that acronym. I am not going to lie. CFS is a bitch and my heart truly goes out to any poor sod that I hear is suffering from it. Unfortunately that is a rather frequent occurrence. I am unbelievably proud to talk about my experience but on average any person I relate my story to knows of someone who has CFS.

In my opinion the root of the illness is stress, plain and simple and the way Western society lives and breathes these days is the culprit. The focus of our living is either centred upon money and people's lack of it, exams that are smothered in pressure to achieve, or the constant presence of the future is forever placed in front of us. There seems to be a hyped up consciousness to plan and secure.

During my recovery I had plenty of time to think about my illness and where it could have originated. I do not claim to have all the answers as I lay blame upon my way of life. It is just odd thoughts that strayed into my mind as I sat very much alone and pondered the demon which had such a tight grip on my life.

I became ill during my A' Levels. I used to be a very neurotic, obsessive person and looking back it seems clear why my body buckled under the enormous pressure I subconsciously put on it. I would not say I wanted to be the best, but I had preconceived, mostly inaccurate, perceptions of what other people and ultimately myself expected of me. The other fundamental factor was that I had no self-belief and hardly any confidence in my own abilities. I also needed fairly high UCAS points to get into a University that I had fallen for on an open day. An overwhelming pressure to succeed was coming at me from many angles. But that is normal for teenagers. Why did I fall prey to an illness that would ultimately deprive me of three years of my life - and not others? The answer is that I internalised all my stress. If I am honest I was completely unaware of all the knots that were so obviously tying up inside me.

My deterioration from a healthy, fit girl to wheelchair user began in the November of 2000 before my final A' Level exams. I pushed myself hard to get through those six months. I would get taxis to school, sleep between lessons in the six-form common area and have very little social life. I made it. I completed my A' Levels and got the necessary grades. I was not in a wheelchair at that time but I did spend the majority of my life lying horizontal in front of the television and crying in desperation if I had to go out. I was just so tired and I didn't know why. I had to defer my place at Sheffield University. My family and I had realised there was no way I could cope in the state I was in. We believed a year's rest would see improvement. It did not.

I returned to my doctor in February 2002 and broke down in tears. I had no energy, I felt fatigued, my muscles hurt and I could not concentrate. I felt drained of strength and had no will to get up in the mornings. I was so tired of being tired. I was in despair because nothing was helping me get better. I did indeed try people's ideas of a wheat-free diet or attempts to build up my strength, but nobody could explain or give me a reason for my condition. That was about to change.

My doctor referred me to a consultant in Essex. I had never heard of a cure for CFS so I blundered in on my first meeting with Dr. David Smith in July 2002 determined I was going off to University that September. Well, DG, as my family came to affectionately call him in private, certainly put an immediate stop to that delusion. For the first time someone could tell me I was ill and why, even if I was not ready to fully comprehend the magnitude of what was happening. I had to give up my life. I was not dying. I had nothing terminal but for the next eighteen months I had to let go of living.

I sat opposite DG, listening to him stripping me of firstly my most pressing dream and ambition of going to University, then to the everyday luxuries of daily existence. I was not allowed to watch television. I was not allowed to read or go on the computer. I was not to listen to music or radio for longer than thirty-minute sessions in hourly intervals. My friends could only visit me one at a time for half an hour per day. I could do ten minutes cross-stitch or drawing per hour. I was to potter. I was to complete limited physical activity, just short walks around the garden. I was to construct my days around 'mindless' activities and of course avoid anything that would cause me stress.

CFS is a biochemical imbalance within the brain brought on by six months or more pre-morbid stress. Certain neurotransmitters are malfunctioning and the brain is not regenerating its energy. DG alerted me to the fact that I was not sleeping properly, that I was catnapping all through the night. My sleeping, or lack of it, was the most important factor to deal with first. Simplistically the recovery programme is about resting the brain both physically and mentally and allowing it time to heal itself. By taking everything away that aggravates it, by doing 'less than you can achieve' you complete the first and perhaps the most imperative stage of recovery. You stop making the illness worse.

Sitting in that chair and hearing my life being stripped down to the bare minimum state of existence threw my mind into a condition of numbness. I could feel my chest tightening as my heart contracted inside me, but it was too soon to digest the enormity of sacrifice I was going to have to make. That came later. There was not a moment to lose though.

I began DG's pacing programme that afternoon and have honestly never looked back since. In my mind there was no choice. DG stated determinedly that he could cure me. The message was that he would not just manage my illness but guide me to full recovery. So the flipside of emotion that I was feeling was pure relief. To have fought against my body so hard for the past year and a half and to be so desperate for the pushing to end, to hear that it was okay to finally give in, lifted the biggest weight I have ever carried on my shoulders.

My voice caught in my throat as I tried to choke back tears when bidding farewell to DG. I would see him again in a month's time but in one way I could breathe again. He had given me the first glimmer of an end to being a captive in my own body.

Now came the hard part, acceptance. DG said to me as I left him that I had to go away and grieve for I was losing something. I had just lost my life. He assured me it would not be forever but I could not know that. All I knew is that I had watched all my friends go off to University from the confines of my bedroom. It really did pinch.

Most of my friends were amazing. Some did not know how to deal with it, which is fair enough, but others visited me regularly and would leave when they knew our time was up. Becky would even bring me Meatball Subs from Subway so we could have lunch together and Hattie would write to me regularly (possibly giving me more information than I cared to hear some times, just joking hun). She kept me up to date with everything going on in her life and still made me feel a part of it. I do not feel it is over the top to describe it as a real lifeline.

I was given so much love and support from my family as well. My Dad was the sturdy, practical provider. He would always bring me things to occupy me within my limitations. My older brother sacrificed his loud music and the freedom to have friends to stay without complaint and I fully appreciated the fact that he never questioned that the television would have to be turned off as I walked into the room for dinner. Finally I shall mention my mum, who was my one companion through it all. She would sit with me every evening reading out the news, weather, sport and film reports off teletext. She gave up a lot of things too, just so I would not have to sit upstairs alone.

Despite all this though, that was the overriding sensation - I felt completely alone. This was my fight. No one could really understand.

It was all on me. No matter how much she wished it my mother could not kiss my forehead and make everything better like she did when I was young. I had honestly never been so scared in all my life. I was absolutely terrified. I was terrified of not being able to cope and most significantly of the recovery programme not working. Somehow though you just have to get a grip on the intensity of emotion erupting inside you. You know that somehow you have to wake up each morning and find the strength in your tired body to get out of bed. The human instinct to survive kicks in and you just get on with it.

The alarm was always on for the same time and I had a specific bedtime. It was about my body enjoying a good eight hours sleep so my brain could start healing and regenerating energy ready for me to use the next day. My doctor tried to explain the condition as 'abnormal normality'. Take the example of a 'normal, healthy person' going skiing. He would spend a day on the slopes and totally exhaust himself. He would go to bed, and the next day, though his muscles would hurt, he would have regenerated his energy supply and could theoretically do the same again. The more exercise he did, the fitter he would get.

CFS sufferers are the complete opposite. I would completely exhaust myself, not sleep properly, not regenerate, so the next day I would have no 'fuel' and would embark upon a dwindling spiral of fatigue. The more I would do, the worse I would feel and the more my condition would deteriorate. That is why it is so abnormal, because anyone feeling in this state is driven by the instinct to fight it and push harder to snap himself out of it. It is kind of ironic I suppose.

My existence became incredibly monotonous and boring. So another emotion to deal with is that of frustration. Escapism is not possible as films, television and books are out of bounds, so you have what seems like an eternity to sit and think about the pathetic weakling you feel you have become.

My grieving took a little longer to hit me. It was about two or three months into the programme but then I literally cried non-stop for a month. I could not help it and I could not control it. I just wept all the time. It made me realise that I wanted someone to talk to though.

I felt I needed someone to whom I could spew out all the shit that was relentlessly bouncing around in my head, without the (unfounded) guilt of upsetting those closest to me. I asked to see a counsellor.

Now I understand that counsellors do not suit everyone but I cannot recommend the experience enough. My hourly sessions were always with Amanda, in the same room at the same time. For six months that was my refuge. I had the comfort that no matter what went on during the week, that was my time to release and not hold back. Some sessions would be gruelling and what emerged sometimes surprised me. I do not know how she did it because for all intents and purposes she just sat and listened, occasionally probing but she managed to draw so much emotion out of me.

Most significantly I acknowledged to myself that I was no longer afraid of death, not even of dying, for I knew pain. Pain so acute I could barely breathe. Pain so acute I actually begged the night to take away my breath. I comforted myself by thinking that no matter how much pain confronted me in life and no matter how grievous the transition would be between life and death, I would be granted with the most precious of states…peace, inner peace. A state I did not believe I would ever discover in life. So I decided that when my time came I would depart with a smile, for I would know that eternal rest would be waiting for me.

Amanda was surprised when she asked me what I wanted as she did not expect to receive the reply that I longed to rest. My point was that I just wanted it to end. It was like a torture. Everyday I had to get up and endure the same monotony. I had to cope with relentless thoughts plaguing my mind, as there was nothing else to occupy it. I was dormant. The pain is like nothing else I have ever experienced. Intense, acute hurt right at my very core of being. It consumed me, drained me of my strength, fight and will. I would cower on the floor clutching my chest and attempt to howl to try to release the pressure I could feel within me. No noise would fill the room though. I had no breath behind the will to scream, for the pain was constricting in my chest.

The fight to get better is the biggest challenge I have ever had to face. The hardest part of that was having to sit in my wheelchair. DG wanted me out of the house. He wanted me to go on holiday and sit somewhere in the sun. He did not want me dwelling on an ill lifestyle at home. There was only one way to manage all that. It was to admit that I had been reduced from a fit and healthy girl who used to go to two hour long dancing lessons on a Saturday afternoon, to a CFS sufferer who could walk no more than about twenty-five metres without enduring extreme fatigue.

I had never felt so humiliated than when my closest friends and family would wheel me round to my local high street in a fucking chair. I would dread seeing people I knew because I was so utterly ashamed of what I had become. It hurt so much because I felt like the illness had beaten me. It had whipped me from inside and pummelled me mercilessly into submission. I hated the fact that I had let it do that to me and I hated myself for allowing it to happen. Ironically improvement followed after swallowing my pride because I finally accepted how ill I actually was. I was ill. I had CFS. That acknowledgement gave me the strength not to let it win. I sat in that wheelchair, baring the excruciating pain because I was taking control. It was simply part of my recovery

The improvement came after about a year when, ever so gradually, DG advised me to start increasing my activity. It was time to push my body slightly. I had to ease the boundaries then allow my brain to get used to the new level of activity and continue to regenerate and then push it further. After a year of being told how little I could do, it was a struggle to find the confidence to push my body. The line 'to get better you cannot feel well' resonated in my head. I was so tired of feeling ill but if this was the final push then bring it on. It was time to kick my illness up the arse.

Though it was six months of true trepidation as I literally found my feet again my progress to fitness was steady. I began with walking a little way then resorting to my wheelchair and gradually the distances lengthened. I built up the visual side with what started as ten minutes here and there of Wimbledon tennis, which grew into catching up on missed episodes of 'Friends' to the ultimate of getting to watch the second 'Lord of the Rings' instalment, 'The Two Towers' that I had missed when it was released in the cinema. I cannot really comment on the emotion I felt through this time, as I am struggling to remember. The progress was so gradual I think that I kept forgetting how far I had come.

Looking back, I can see it now. Immense pride and relief may be the best words to describe my state when DG discharged me in the late summer of 2004. Also, of course gratitude. I am not sure there is any point in mincing words. DG gave me my life back and I think he knows through treating so many people over the years and after receiving my card just how thankful I am to him. DG, you almost hold the rank of God in my mind, quite frankly.

I started Sheffield University in 2004, three years after I was initially supposed to begin my English Language with Linguistics course. I was still building my strength up when I first arrived. I was fully fit but I just did not quite have the stamina to party like my flatmates. It did not take long to catch up.

I love studying at Sheffield. It has certainly surpassed my expectations and given the fact that I had three years to build it up, that certainly says something. I took major advantage of everything my first year had to offer, in particular enjoying the fact I could finally live my youth.

Outside of study, clubbing and alcohol abuse I also wrote for the student newspaper, in which I was invited to attend a sex goddess lesson, went on a blind date for Valentine's Day and attended a preliminary G8 meeting in Derby. I performed in a production of 'The Vagina Monologues' and took part in one off volunteering days organised through the University. I did not just go to University, I sucked it dry of all the fun I had the energy to take part in. I fucking lived it!

I am now about to head back for my second year at the age of twenty-two, after having spent seven weeks doing voluntary conservation work in Chile. I felt I had to do something over my summer break, for now I have my energy back I cannot sit still. I feel like I am wasting time.

I was able to finally lay ghosts to rest in Chile. The majority of my time was spent in a place called Namoncahue. It is a mountain range and I lived in a small cabana two and a half hours trek up a mountain away from civilisation. I loved the experience. In particular the opportunity to sit in the open, surrounded by the forest and mountain range, closing my eyes and hearing silence, allowing me to feel a taster of that inner peace. For the only stresses that confronted our team of eleven up there was whether we had chopped enough wood for the next morning's fire or whether too much snow would fall to prevent us from working. A slight difference in paradigm compared to the strict 'nine to five' work consciousness of my culture.

I trekked up mountains with a heavy rucksack on my back, I worked each day carrying out tasks such as sawing, chopping wood, carrying logs, building and fully enjoying feeling my muscles really work hard. I did indeed get to stick my middle finger up to the illness that consumed me for so many years. I realised sitting there in freedom that I do not answer to it anymore. I need not think of it when I am tired. Never again will it plague my thoughts and never again will it be the first thing I think of when my body is weary. I am well. I will never again wake in fear of it or worry about its possible return.

I now find it hard to communicate the intensity of my feeling. It is the complete opposite end of the scale compared to the pain I endured. It is beyond happiness or relief. It is complete exhilaration and excitement for the life that I can live. Right now it's almost as though I am on a constant high. Now, whenever there is a challenge, I want to face it head on, for my mentality is "what is the worst that could happen?"

I love to push my body and feel it working. I love to be reminded of the difference between my muscles wasting away and lying dormant. I love the jerk as my heart starts pounding blood through my body; feeling the adrenaline kicking in, seeping into my veins and pounding exhilaration to my very core. I like to feel my hands shaking, the dryness in my mouth and barely feeling in control. I love it when my mind becomes a mess as a mash of dizziness blinds my eyes to the monotonous shit of the ordinary. I am addicted to feeling the systematic impulses of energy surging through my muscles, making me feel as powerful as the mother fucking son of a bitch that put us all on this Earth. I love the tingles in my stomach and the heat swelling around my heart as it lets me know that I am truly alive. Chile really allowed me to feel all that.

I do not regret being ill. I look on it as an experience that catapulted my view on life into a new perspective. My travels to Chile shifted it again but it has been the single most important event to happen to me in my young life and has shaped my life to come. I have shed a skin, but the scar will never let me forget those three years of dormancy, which is both my strength and weakness, my good fortune and my worst, my wisdom and my form of blindness, my gratitude and my anger, my heart and my soul.

What scares me slightly now is becoming caught in the trap again. Allowing the stresses of everyday life in our society to suck me in and consume me once more. CFS is the manifestation of all the unnecessary stresses that we put on ourselves. The very fact though that I am aware of the illness's origin equips me with the confidence that I will never allow it to haunt me again.

Right now, I have no thoughts of mortgages or providing for the future. Right now it is time for me to live. What excites me right now is *not* knowing what I am going to do. I am going to just enjoy waiting and taking advantage of whatever opportunities I can make happen. I cannot wait to see where I end up or what will happen next but I know full well I shall enjoy the ride to the utmost and never let anything pass me by.

I feel stronger for having had and overcome CFS and I certainly would not change my past, even if I had that impossible luxury. I would not possess the inner strength and wisdom that I feel gives me the confidence to tackle anything life dares to throw at me, without that illness. I would not be the stubborn cow, whom I discovered in Chile, that I am actually secretly so proud of. I would not have released my passionate nature that insists I give 100% to everything I do. What would be the point in offering anything less? I love my unique perspective on life now. I view the world so differently to most people and I consider it as one of my greatest assets.

CFS caused me pain, but it also gave me the overwhelming excitement of being alive. From shadow comes pain, but with light comes strength and wisdom. I lay to rest my friend and nemesis. Cheers and farewell.

Most useful aid to recovery - Dr David Smith

Recommended websites
www.me-cfs-recovery.co.uk
www.me-cfs-treatment.com
www.ayme.org.uk
www.afme.org.uk

Lizzie Neal

David's story

We must practise prevention and say *no* if doing too much. Many in retrospect have been doing too much for years before becoming ill!

When I look back over my life, I realise that there may have been some precursors to my CFS/ME. I was a full-term baby weighing three and half ounces in 1941. As a baby I had a recurrent metabolic acidosis and iron deficiency anaemia. As a child I pushed myself, although I learned to develop stamina. At the age of twelve I had measles and unknowingly exercised vigorously whilst incubating it. It was after that that symptoms of CFS/ME occurred on and off, and as a result I was off school for a whole term.

CFS/ME is a condition where relapses are common, and there have been periods in my life when I have felt absolutely fine and periods where I have been seriously ill. The next illness started when I was fourteen years old and it lasted throughout a whole term at school. I had recurrent bronchitis, the only attacks of asthma in my life, and pneumonia, twice. My immune system must have been under a lot of strain.

When I was working for, and during my 'O' Levels, (standard grade as it is called now), I had what I would now call 'Brain Fog,' and my performance dropped dramatically. The school doctor discovered my recurrent low blood sugar and consequently I carried around a jar of sugar and was allowed to get tea in the kitchen. Six spoonfuls of sugar temporarily restored me!

As time went on I became more and more tired physically and mentally. I would rest and pace myself during the holidays, be fine for the first few weeks of the term, and then suddenly go down- hill. The final insult was the school doctor, with great insight for the 1950's, forbidding me from playing games or running. I had to take a gentle walk! You can imagine what the other boys thought as I had no obvious physical injury, like a leg in plaster! I have since realised that this is a very common problem for people with CFS or the more severe version ME, because, except for an episodic facial pallor, they may not look ill at all.

Pacing myself did help and I will always remember Dr Clelland, the school doctor, giving me such support and kindness. He did a very important thing, he used to sit me down and get me to explain exactly what I felt was happening, how my stamina was and so on. Later, he told me that when I felt faint I should see the matron and go to bed early. That would temporarily restore me. In retrospect this may have been the beginning of the neurally mediated hypotension, which is more severe than mere postural hypotension. In neurally mediated hypotension the blood drains away from the head so that areas of the brain have inadequate circulation and the symptoms vary depending on which parts of the brain are affected. This is why 'brain fog' occurs.

The next stage was my first year at medical school. I developed what was labelled 'Atypical Glandular Fever,' but I remember my father writing to the haematologist saying that whatever it was, it couldn't be glandular fever, because the tests were negative. On the other hand my spleen was very enlarged - so what was it? Later I even had angina when running.

My father died in 1964 when I was a second year medical student. This was obviously a difficult time for me and my illness started to re-occur. One day I fainted on a ward round. And later as a resident, when I was looking after some neurology patients, I caught a viral infection from a patient who came in as an emergency, and over the next few weeks found my concentration and physical stamina decreasing.

My next residency was in surgery and I was looking after some patients in the Corstorphine Hospital, as our own unit in Edinburgh Royal Infirmary was being re-furbished. One night I was called to see a patient at 2am. I saw him - and later only remembered going to wash my hands. A nurse, who came to see why I hadn't returned to the nursing station, had found me unconscious. I was put to bed in my room and observed by the night superintendent. I only responded to painful stimuli and was apparently unconscious for five hours, being transferred to a ward in the

Royal Infirmary the following day. That episode was later labelled as 'having had a severe faint'. However, the night superintendent, with years of experience in what today would be called high-dependency care, told me that she had never seen a five hour faint before! (Often with CFS/ME, the symptoms are there, but the doctor plays them down because he can't relate them to any known condition).

In retrospect, this was the first really bad attack of my neurally mediated hypotension. Neurally mediated hypotension is why CFS/ME patients have decreased brain circulation. This is why the patient, the family, and above all, the physician, must look out for, and enquire about, recurrent facial pallor. This is what I call 'The Facial Pallor Sign.' When it is present the underlying brain circulation is decreased, often including decreased circulation to the hypothalamus and the pituitary glands and then extra strain on the adrenal glands.

When I finished my residency I took sick leave, returning to work part time for three months. During this time I wondered what was wrong with me, especially as I found I couldn't remember things I had read and had difficulty with people's names - which is the one thing I have to work on even today! In fact, from that date, I was never able to take a higher medical examination, and, in particular, multiple choice papers were very confusing to me.

Throughout the 1970s and 1980s, trying my best to work in medical general practice, I had periods of what seemed like depression, and I was needing an increasing amount of rest at weekends. From the mid-1970's onwards I found that I was feeling more and more tired and when we went on holiday in 1976 to Granton-on-Spey in the Highlands of Scotland, I tried playing golf. This meant that I had to spend most of my time between meals resting in my hotel bedroom.

Between 1970 and 1980 I worked full-time in North Berwick. This meant working as part of a team. At first I was known for my ability to dictate a letter with no mistakes and get through my administrative duties quickly, however, this situation gradually deteriorated. Sequencing, that is, putting thoughts and tasks into an order, is a particular problem for many CFS/ME sufferers, and certainly something I had difficulty with. I also became much more tired. I needed more and more rest at weekends and our social life went totally by the board – except for my mother, my sister and a very close family friend, who demonstrated what real friendship and support really is.

I continued to deteriorate and my resistance to infections decreased. A consultant urologist diagnosed chronic prostatitis and had me on the antibiotic, Septrin, for six months. In January 1980 I had to resign from the North Berwick Practice as I realised that I was not going to get better with the heavy medical work load, and nights and weekends on call. In those days the population of North Berwick doubled during the summer months. For two months during the Summer of 1979 there were only two GP's to cover the whole town, as well as the holiday makers! One of the two was me! We were so short staffed that each of us was on call every second night and either Saturday or Sunday at weekends.

The inevitable result of this was that one Friday, at the end of the summer of 1979, I went to bed and was literally unable to get up again. At first I thought there was a neurological problem, and, in retrospect there was, and it was due to ME. I use that name to differentiate it from what I see as a milder version or variant, namely Chronic Fatigue Syndrome. I had various neurological symptoms, including right foot drop (I was unable to hold my foot straight), fasciculations, and clonus, all which are also found in conditions such as MS, which is why CFS/ME is so often misdiagnosed. My balance had gone, I had terrible headaches and muscle pain, and I wasn't able to write with my right hand. Initially I had six weeks in bed.

I did feel depressed, but this was a reactive depression secondary to my incapacity and illness. At times I wondered if perhaps it was depression, but luckily for me I had the medical knowledge and training to be able to realise that the depression was only a *part* of what was going on. I was helped greatly by the late Dr Richard Parry, a psychiatrist, who supported me and listened while we tried to work out what was really happening. Together we diagnosed CFS/ME in 1981.

I can understand why medical colleagues, and especially psychiatrists, have mistaken CFS/ME for depression. This is due to a lack of awareness of the many symptoms of CFS/ME which can mimic psychiatric or psychosomatic illness. Many people with a severe illness develop a reactive or secondary depression, as a result of not being able to work, chronic pain and so on, but it is *not the cause* of the illness. Just as someone can have a reactive depression to cancer. In computer terms: *depression* is as if the person is running a software programme that makes him or her think in negative ways. *CFS/ME* is as if they have *decreased power* to the computer, so that the software will not run properly. This is what we call 'Brain Fog' today. However, it is important to understand that on-going negative life events, recurrent infections, chronic inflammation and so on, can and does depress the immune system, and if the individual is worried or trying to do too much, their 'fight or flight' stress response can also get turned on.

When I got back to a certain level I did some locums, working part-time as a principal GP for ten years, from 1980 until 1990. With the medical ignorance of the time I tried to carry on working under cover of medication. I was given twelve amitriptyline 25mg tabs daily to suppress my headaches and eight Co-proxamol tablets daily to suppress the muscle pain. In reality all this did was allow the CFS/ME to continue in a masked state. In 1990 I tried to increase my workload and became very ill. After six months of being unable to work at all, I was given early retirement on health grounds from the first of January 1990, when I was aged fifty.

At that point I decided it was my responsibility to get myself better. This would be my priority. There would be time for work when I got myself better.

ME destroyed fifteen years of my life and that of my wife Jennifer as well. It decreased the quality of life of the whole family. Throughout this period I was unable to look after myself, and was totally reliant on the support that Jennifer gave me. It is essential to give enough support to families. Many professionals don't realise the devastating effect that CFS/ME has on the whole family unit, and as a result, inadequate support is often given by the GP and the social services, including Disability Benefits.

Having retired from the health service on health grounds, and having made the decision that if I was going to get better I would have to find the answers for myself, initially my focus was on finding a way to restore myself to health. Later I extended this to helping, and learning with, people who had CFS/ME. Today, we must concentrate on how we prevent people getting CFS/ME in the first place and on early diagnosis and treatment. Help must be given especially to the most ill, the 25% with ME who can be ill for years, and also the children.

The biggest milestone in my process of recovery was in 1990 when I took the decision 'if it is to be, it's up to me' because, to my frustration, I realised that nobody else knew what to do. I realised that 'responsibility is the ability to respond' and I nurtured a burning belief that someday I would get better.

My recovery started with developing my insights, knowledge, and the skills to apply them. That is what I did. As soon as I got myself up and about in January 1990 I went to see a psychiatrist in the Edinburgh Royal Infirmary. He thought I seemed very positive about the illness. It was because I knew I could work to get better. He seemed impressed by my attitude towards recovery and I never needed to go back. I had been using cognitive therapy techniques with my own patients since

1976 and so I had some of the knowledge I needed to help myself to keep positive.

The use of the alpha state helped enormously. This is a healing state which enables your body and mind to heal itself. You can teach yourself the alpha state, or learn it with the help of a qualified practitioner. Modifying the frequency of your brain waves and entering the alpha state places you in direct communication with your subconscious mind and the rest of your body. It produces a healing state described by Dr. Benson, the cardiologist who heads Harvard University's Mind-Body Institute, as the 'relaxation response'. This is the exact opposite of the 'fight or flight' Response. I joined the British Society of Medical and Dental Hypnosis, and learned self-hypnosis, deep meditation, and autogenic training, and I used those for mind-body healing.

When I was assessed by a reflexologist friend she said that I was healed in mind but not yet in body. At the time I did not understand what she was getting at. I was on a journey, learning new insights and new ways of doing things. As I now understand, *healing* actually begins in the quantum field, and *illness* begins there as too, years before it begins in the physical. Healing then starts with a change of attitude - the individual stops being 'poor me' or a victim and at whatever level takes back control, thus the change in mind leads to a change in the mental, emotional, and then the physical state.

What the reflexologist picked up on was the toxicity and the inflammation still present in my body at that time. I continued using the alpha state and then later I worked on detoxification using the antioxidant 'Revenol', to rid me of pesticide (this was used at Chernobyl). I also used the Australian probiotic, 'Prime Directive', initially for my gut, and also producing improvement in my blood as shown with Light Phase microscopy.

At the same time I had to learn to pace myself and realised that '*if you do not use it you lose it.*' Unfortunately, just as with a sports injury, if you overuse it you can also lose it. In April 1990 it took five minutes at worst to go up a flight of stairs holding on with two hands. I made a decision that before the end of the summer I would get to the top of

North Berwick Law Hill, which is five hundred feet up. At that time I could walk three hundred yards on the level. I paced myself, so if it was a good day, I would follow the same route but extend it by fifteen or twenty yards. If it was a really bad day, and I was decompensated I didn't even try to go out. (When a person compensates they are able to keep going even when they are not feeling well, decompensating happens where a person's compensating abilities have become exhausted and they are suddenly no longer able to compensate). I was like an athlete pacing myself. Before the end of July 1990, my eldest daughter and I went with a camera, and she took a picture of me on the top of the North Berwick Law Hill.

However, 'graded exercise' and cognitive therapy only got me back to 70% of my previous physical and mental level. They, by themselves, were only a part of the answer, and by themselves only work well for the least unwell 20% of patients. With those alone I would never have got back to full time work as I did. There were still several things I had to do. Cognitive trials appear to exclude people with perceived mental problems (which in reality can be due to poor circulation of the limbic system) and completely ignore the physical side with the decreased circulation to the hypothalamus and the pituitary. In the over three hundred patients I have studied in detail, many were excluded from cognitive trials on psychiatric grounds or because they lacked motivation or were labelled as not co-operating! Also often excluded were those who were unable to attend as outpatients, because they were house bound or bed-ridden.

Insights for improving mental and physical function were: how to be aware when initially de-compensating and to take rest at the right point; how to treat neurally-mediated hypotension and brain circulation with minute doses of nimodipine, dowsing these precise doses; how to treat brain function with nutrition; how to detoxify the brain of neurotoxins, and body fat and muscle of chemical toxicity; how to treat mineral deficiency in CFS/ME; how to boost the immune system in CFS/ME; how to rid the gut of candida and parasites; long term dealing with any remaining infection – viral or bacterial; how to maximise the quality of the diet for best health; how to use the alpha state and visualisation and other techniques; cognitive and related techniques were used when the patient had a brain circulation good enough to understand and apply them; physical rehabilitation techniques appropriate to the state of the patient and never forcing them to do too much.

The toxicity in my case was caused by organophosphates. I have a genetic susceptibility to them. Different people have different susceptibilities. That is, CFS/ME does not hit everyone in the same way. I learned how to dowse and avoid things that were not good for me.

In 1995 I was bitten by an insect on the chest in Jamaica whilst on holiday. I immediately went back to my hotel room and cleaned it with antiseptic. The causal infection was definitely bacterial clinically, but the type was never decided. When I got back I had to be rushed to the Royal Infirmary, to a unit I had previously worked on, because I had five abscesses in my liver. In fact my immune system at that time was virtually non-existent! If it had not been for modern medicine and technology and superb care I would be dead. However, it is important to remember that although modern medicine is a wonderful fire brigade, it is far better not to start the fire in the first place! During that period I was given two antibiotics by drip, and the abscesses were drained under a scanner. I was unable to work for six months. After that, I resumed my own private practice and workshops.

I was Hon. Medical Officer of Edinburgh MESH (CFS/ME Self Help Group) for about twelve years, retiring by mutual agreement when I was sixty-six. The committee did and do tremendous work on support and disability benefits, and some worked very well on relaxation and even their lifestyle. But many have the crucial lack of belief that they can get better. In everyone I have seen who has really become better, there has been a burning desire that someday they will get better. They may not know how or when, but they start the journey. For best results there is also help by some family members, friends, and a good supportive family doctor. It is the same with patients who have spontaneous remission and recovery from inoperable or officially untreatable cancer.

I became the Medical Director of Equilibrium Associates Limited, which is a company working in the areas of stress management and corporate health and performance as well as increasing energy. I worked full time, running workshops in stress and lifestyle management, as well as seeing patients on a one-to-one basis, and now, at the age of sixty-six years, I am still giving workshops and seeing patients part-time.

In the last five years I have become interested in Energy Medicine and what happens in the quantum field. Some Japanese researchers call CFS/ME 'Reduced Total Body Electric Charge Syndrome', in which the chi, now becoming scientifically measurable, is reduced in the young CFS/ME patient to that of someone in their upper eighties. No wonder one feels so tired. I have even learned Reiki - something which years ago I would never have believed in. I have also learned how to get rid of all past negative emotions, how to forgive myself and everyone and everything else, and how to have high emotional intelligence in each present moment. I came from a Scottish culture and religious background of over sixty years ago, so learning to love myself and not to be judgemental, is very important. The focus had to be on the present and on the future with no complaining about the past. Thinking in purpose is about thinking what you are actually trying to do and achieve in that moment in time. The longest journey begins with a single step and is carried out a bit at a time. Let go of all the dramas of the past and live in the now.

In summary we have to learn to have an open mind, to look at *new* ways of doing things, *new* paradigms of thought, whilst also continuing to advance conventional medicine. It is the *holistic whole* that is important. We must treat the causes, not wait for the effects. The causes develop first in the quantum field years before they even appear as mental emotional or physical symptoms. Also we must practice prevention, which is what most of my work is about today.

Recommended books
"Clinical and Scientific Basis of Myalgic Encephalomyelitis/Chronic Fatigue Syndrome" by Jay A. Goldstein (Author, Editor), Byron M. Hyde (Author, Editor), Nightingale Research Foundation (Corporate Author), P. H. Levine (Editor)

"Betrayal by the Brain: Neurological Basis of Chronic Fatigue Syndrome, Fibromyalgia Syndrome and Related Neural Network Disorders" (The Haworth Library ... Networks in Health & Illness +) by Jay Goldstein (author)

"The Power of Now: A Guide to Spiritual Enlightenment" by Eckhart Tolle

"Your Erroneous Zones: Step-by-step Advice for Escaping the Trap of Negative Thinking and Taking Control of Your Life" by Wayne W. Dyer

Recommended websites
www.cfids-me.org/aacfs/ (American Association for Chronic Fatigue Syndrome)
www.freespace.virgin.net/david.axford/melist.htm (ME/CFS List of Medical Articles)
www.meassociation.org.uk/content/view/114The ME Association & Article from the Times)

David's advice - become your own expert, keep an open mind, get support, and find what works for you. Be holistic and use the best of international conventional medicine and complimentary medicine, including remedial nutrition.

Dr David Mason Brown

Jess's story

A raw food diet helped me beat CFS

It was Monday morning and as usual I didn't feel awake enough to get out of bed. In fact, my body still felt like it was the middle of the night. I lay there as my body ached all over and my eyes struggled to open. I knew it must have been about 8am, because the light shone in through the curtains and I could hear my university flatmates getting ready for lectures. I told myself "it's Monday morning and everyone feels like this on a Monday morning"- but I'd been getting the 'Monday morning feeling' everyday for the last two weeks. I was starting to get behind with my university work and my lecturers told me that I had to go to see the college doctor if I wanted an extension. Knowing I had to leave the house in time for my doctor's appointment I sat up in bed, only to lie straight back down again. I felt like death warmed up. I had felt pretty grim for the last two weeks, but nowhere near as bad as this. I couldn't even sit up without nearly passing out.

An hour passed and I still didn't feel any better. I tried to cancel my doctor's appointment but they couldn't fit me in for another two weeks. I knew that would be too late for the coursework deadline so I had no choice but to drag myself there. When I arrived, the doctor seemed a bit short with me and pushed for time. He asked me what my problem was and three minutes later I was being ushered out his office with a prescription for anti-depressants. I tried to explain how I felt and that I was by no means depressed. Sure, I didn't feel my normal self, but who would with zero energy levels? He made it quite clear that he was the expert and feeling so weak and ill, I wasn't in a position to argue.

I called my mum outside the surgery and she ordered me to rip up the prescription whilst I was on the phone to her. It did cross my mind to try the drugs. I felt so out of sorts and wanted to get on with my life, but I'm so thankful I didn't because it's so much better to treat the cause, not just the symptoms, no matter how bad the problem seems to be.

A few months went by and I didn't seem to be getting any better. Whenever I had a good day, the next day I would feel burned out and back to square one. My average day was spent in bed drifting in and out of sleep and taking paracetamol around the clock. If I knew there was somewhere I had to go, I would spend a couple of days saving up my energy to prepare for it.

I was in a two year relationship with Nick at the time. Every Thursday his Dad's television show 'Parkinson' was recorded. I knew it meant a lot to Nick for me to be there, so I would drag myself into the waiting car, watch the show all spaced out, and then feel like curling up in the green room afterwards, as everyone enjoyed the hospitality around me.

One day I was called into a meeting with the head of my course, who was quite a firm man. We needed to discuss why I was getting so behind. I honestly thought that he was about to withdraw me from the course as I had heard he had previously asked five students to leave on the grounds of absent coursework. I sat down in his office and to my utter amazement it turned out that he had been suffering from CFS for twenty years. He went from being hard faced to all smiles as soon as I blurted out my condition. He was very kind and helpful and we talked for about an hour and a half. He told me not to worry and to hand in course work whenever I could - which was a far cry from what I was expecting him to say! I had to see the college doctor every month to satisfy the university board. Every time it was the same three minute routine without fail. Enter doctor's office. Briefly sit down. Explain my ailments. Be prescribed anti-depressants. Try and argue. Leave office. Rip up prescription. Go home.

I became a vegetarian when I was ten years old because one of my best friends had declared herself 'meat-free'. However, at university I had a flat-mate who made my life hell for it. He was abusive and called me names, and encouraged his friends to call me names. It was so upsetting that one day it became too much and I went back to meat for the first time in eight years. I went on to eat meat for a full year, before I discovered my 'ten magic foods'.

One day the Big Breakfast TV crew paid a visit to our university. They wanted me and some students to take part in a game show that would be transmitted live across the UK. It involved getting three students' parents live on the phone to see how well they knew us. My mum and eldest brother, Ben, answered their questions correctly about me and after a manic supermarket sweep style raid on another student's bedroom to bring back ten listed items, and with the kind help of Richard Bacon, I finally did it. My prize was a year's supply of Baked Beans!

My CFS was at its worst in my second year of university. I was really ill and would drag myself between university in Birmingham, my home in Buckinghamshire, and Nick's place in Berkshire - although he was very busy running the celebrity restaurant he had just set up with his father. When I was really frail I stayed at home with my fantastic family looking after me, where I spent much of my time. When I was in Birmingham I never had the energy to do any cooking and we all ate at different times. Funnily enough it was for this reason that I would just eat my vegetables in their raw state, along with fruit and a pot of hummus. Over a period of time I noticed changes in my energy levels and improvements in my overall state of health. I could stay out of bed longer in the day and my head would feel clearer. I began craving a simple diet of no more than ten foods, consisting of bananas, satsumas, apples, mangos, broccoli, carrots, cucumber, mini sweet corn, bean sprouts and hummus. Whenever I ate these foods I would see improvement, whereas other food such as bread, pasta and milk chocolate left me physically hurting in pain, and so fatigued. It's not that these ten foods are necessarily superior to any other raw fruit or vegetables, just that my body could digest them more easily so I had energy left for my body to begin the self healing process.

The doctor at home was slightly more caring than the one at university. He only prescribed me anti-depressants three times instead of the college doctor's six times! He tested me for coeliac disease, a condition where the body is allergic to the protein in wheat, known as gluten. I was told that the test may come back negative because you have to have gluten present in the body during the test and I didn't (because by this time I was living on my ten magic foods) so I wasn't surprised when the result came back as negative.

One day, when I was at home in Buckinghamshire sorting through my bookshelf, a green book 'leapt' off the shelf and hit me on the head! It read, 'Raw Energy Recipes by Susanna and Leslie Kenton'. I couldn't believe it! I had bought that book in a car boot sale when I was eight years old but I had never read it, and here it was, just when I had already started healing thanks to my ten magic foods! I read it and was intrigued. This book provided the missing link between why I had started to feel better, and what I had to do to get fully better.

As well as eating a raw food diet, I began to visualise a return to good health. One day when I had been lying in bed watching the London Marathon on television, I decided to make a goal - to run the 26.4 mile marathon myself - once I was better. To help me reach that goal I visualised myself everyday, in superb health, crossing the finishing line. I made myself *feel* what it would be like to finish a marathon - the joy, achievement, accomplishment and more. I visualised deeper and deeper until the hairs on the back of my neck stood on end! It paid off, because a year or so after I had cured myself, I ran the Flora London Marathon in just over four hours.

Although I did make attempts at going back to a cooked vegan diet, I felt tired and my glands swelled up whenever I ate wheat. So today my diet is very different from my university days. As I write this

I am a 100% raw vegan and have been for six years. The raw food way really works for me, and I feel great on it.

My lifestyle is also different. I now live with Tom, my boyfriend, and the joint managing director of the online business I founded when I was twenty-three years old, Total Raw Food Ltd. I felt so passionate about eating raw foods for high energy health that I just had to spread the word. Our house in Brighton is a raw vegan home and there is no cooked food, dairy or meat to be found within. Instead you'll find two fridges full of raw, organic, bio dynamic food; plus massive bowls of fruit and tons of superfoods like Maca, Raw Chocolate, Goji Berries, Mesquite and natural sweetener Raw Agave Nectar to name a few. We have an oven that we use as an extra cupboard. It's never been used as an oven and I don't even know if it works! It just so happened that Tom was already raw when we met, so I was quite fortunate with that.

I eat a raw and living vegan diet intuitively, when I am genuinely hungry, instead of it being because it's breakfast time, lunch time or tea time. I find this approach really sustains my energy levels. I have no toxic food in my diet which will compromise my energy levels or my health, because it's not worth the health price I have to pay for it. I usually start the day with a porridge made from raw oat groats, water, and vanilla essential oil, sweetened with raw agave nectar. I usually have a fruit smoothie daily made with bananas, frozen raspberries, mango and the juice of a freshly squeezed orange. Later on in the day I have a large green mixed salad with seaweed and a raw nut or seed based dressing that I have freshly whizzed up in my powder blender. If I need to snack, I will have fresh fruit or raw chocolate. I drink about three litres of water a day. I used to let myself get dehydrated without realising it, which affected my energy levels. I only use products that are free from dangerous chemicals. I use Raw Gaia living organic skincare on my face and coconut butter as a moisturiser and conditioner, which I leave on overnight. I have recently found a totally natural shampoo called Mistry, which is fabulous. If I can't eat whatever I put on my body then I won't apply it. I try and exercise every day too, but when I am too busy I will do ten minutes of rebounding.

I now work full time with Total Raw Food Ltd, sometimes up to eighteen hours a day! This is something that I could never have imagined myself doing when I was suffering from CFS. I still need more sleep at night than the average raw fooder, at least eight hours per night, whereas many people on a high raw diet can get away with around six hours of sleep. I have gone back to having a busy social life again, and generally feel great and am always up for having fun! Although I do not run as much as I did when I was training for the marathon, I love going on long walks with my black Labrador. When Tom and I went on our first holiday together earlier this year, we rescued a very young puppy that had been dumped and abandoned on a beach. As he is now rapidly growing into a big strong dog, we are looking forward to taking him on beautiful long walks too within the South Downs.

Most useful aid to recovery - raw food diet

Recommended books – "How to Create Your Raw Reality" by Tom Fenton

Recommended websites - www.totalrawfood.com

Jess's advice - The one piece of advice I would give to anyone wanting to beat CFS is to gradually transition yourself onto a high raw diet and slowly eliminate toxic, addictive foods. Throw out any chemical beauty and household products in place of earth and human friendly alternatives from your local health store. Don't think too much about going raw - just go for it. It could be the best decision that you've ever made in your life.

Jess Michael

Bob's Story

The Mantz Straw

I've battled with several 'syndromes' over the past 15 years. I've gone through years of suffering with Chronic Fatigue Syndrome (CFS), irritable bowel syndrome (IBS), insomnia, headaches, leaky gut syndrome, tonsillitis and depression. I could write a full book on all the doctors that I've visited and all the prescriptions that I've taken but I want to keep this as short as possible.

I remember reading the title of a book, 'Sick and Tired of Feeling Sick and Tired' - that would describe exactly how I felt a few years into what I now know to be CFS.

I remember reading about people who had suffered with CFS and who were now feeling better and thinking - there is no way that I am going to get over this. I am not going to feel better. I may as well kill myself now. I cried myself to bed many a night wondering 'why me?' Thankfully I had the love of a strong family and just that thought alone prevented me from taking thoughts of offing myself any further than just thinking about it.

OK – so the short of it is that I got sick a lot growing up. Seemed like I had strep throat or bronchitis once a month. Unfortunately I also had a doctor who loved antibiotics. You may need antibiotics for certain ailments like Streptococcal infections but I have a faint recollection of going for a check up and walking out with a shot of penicillin!

Shots, pills, that great tasting pink antibiotic - I was always on one or the other. It is only now that I can hypothesize that that was a major contributor to my later suffering.

It was November 1987 when I first developed the symptoms that combined to form my CFS. I came down with the 'flu' the first week of November. It was still there two months later. It was still there two years later. Remnants of it were still around fifteen years later. I felt like I had the flu every single day for the next two years. Weakness permeated everything. It wasn't tiredness, it was 'sapped' weakness, the kind you get with the flu. I missed lots of school and had to get a tutor.

I continued seeking all kinds of doctors to try and track down why I felt weak all the time. Internists, allergists, endocrinologists. As for tests, I had positive tests for allergies, so I started on allergy shots, but otherwise everything came back normal. Oh, except for my temperature. I was always running low, 97.5 or so, but that never concerned anyone.

I even saw a counselor and tried prozac and amitryptiline. However, I knew it wasn't depression making me feel like crap. It was feeling like crap that was making me depressed!

I headed to Johns Hopkins Hospital to see the best of the best. My dad took time off from work and drove me down. We met with a doctor for about 45 minutes who thought that I may have had meningitis back in November and that I was probably suffering from a post viral syndrome that would correct itself by the prom in May. It didn't. A few months went by. Every minute of every day I felt weak. Not one day passed that I didn't feel crappy. I was now into my second year of weakness. Depression was growing. Sick and tired, sick and tired …

I wound up at an Ear, Nose and Throat specialist. I had a deviated septum that was causing sinus infections. The septum was re-broken and reset but within three months it had begun to pull back out of place. The surgery didn't take. I later found out that this locally famous doctor had been suspended for crack use. What a joke. Found myself at a second ENT. Guess what? I had chronic tonsillitis and they had to come out. I started to get far fewer sore throats and I did have a day or two in a few months when my weakness subsided. I actually knew what it felt like to feel good again. The only problem was that the day or two that I started to feel better actually served as a horrible 'tease' as I would slip back into weakness. I would have a day or two of relief and then weeks of relapse.

I also had this enjoyable urge to faint when I got up quickly. Once I even fell through a glass coffee table after getting up from reading comics. Joy, Joy.

I went to see a local internist. I was now approaching three years of sickness. He diagnosed me with CFS. Finally. I felt a little better just hearing that I had a name for this demon.

I also underwent a scope because I had also been experiencing severe stomach pains and bouts of diarrhoea over the last year. He diagnosed my IBS and prescribed metamucil. It worked. My IBS was lessened tremendously, probably around 80%. Most importantly, the pain was lessened and inadvertently my doctor had turned me on to natural healing. If a simple product containing psyllium could cure something as well as a drug could - what else was out there?

I had read Durk Pearson and Sandy Shaw's book 'Life Extensions' a few years back and that drew me to nutrition. Consequently I joined the Life Extension Foundation. Here is what I did directly because of Durk and Sandy: I used L-Tryptophan while it was still available. And it worked well for my insomnia. I took Life Extension mix which is a very high dose of multi-vitamin and mineral supplement. I also took other nutritional products like Ginseng, Co-Enzyme Q10 and DHEA.

During the next year I tried acupuncture, hypnosis and self-hypnosis. I also tried all vegetarian and vegan diets but they didn't work out for me.

I used melatonin in combination with the old adage, "Early to bed, early to rise." I went to bed at 9pm and was up no later than 6am. I later learned that that is a golden rule for insomniacs - get up at exactly the same time every day regardless of how little sleep you got the night before. Eventually the body will force you to sleep the next night. It's a tough thing to do when you've perhaps just fallen asleep 15 minutes before the alarm clock rings - but do it. Get up. That, combined with the melatonin, worked like a charm.

I started to read Dr. Weil and made some changes to my overall lifestyle. I bought a set of weights and exercised. It was extremely difficult. Dr Weil said that it will suck. It will hurt. You will feel like someone socked you in the gut. And it did. It was so tough to work through all that. But I had to. I worked out three times a week or so with the weights and it paid off. A few weeks into that routine and I had my first full week of feeling good.

I transferred into New Jersey's Trenton State College the following year and graduated in 1994. Just a short seven years ago I had been happy to make it to the next day, and here I was a college graduate. I owe that first to my family, second to Durk and Sandy and the Life Extension Foundation, and finally to the doctors who did name what I had.

The problem with finishing college was - where the hell could I work? Yeah, seven to eight days in a row of feeling good was great in the big scheme of things, but that wouldn't cut it in a nine to five world. Can you imagine telling your boss, "Yeah, I'll be calling out sick the next twenty-eight days. See you next month." I couldn't handle a full time corporate gig.

Fortunately both my parents are educators. I became a substitute teacher. The hours were good and I could be 'off-call' as needed. I did this for about four years.

One thing that had always gnawed at me was my low body temperature. I read and re-read Durk's description of his undiagnosed thyroid issues and his use of Armour Thyroid. I purchased Broda Barnes' book, 'Hypothyroidism, The Unsuspected Illness.' It is one book that I have read several times, again and again. After reading this book I was convinced that he was writing about me. I bought a thermometer and took my basal temperature. You keep a shaken down thermometer by your bed and stick it under your arm as soon as you awaken with as little movement as possible. A temperature lower than 98 indicates a sluggish thyroid. As expected it was low. Now I had to find a doctor who would diagnose and treat by that method. After all, all my blood work always came back normal. The Broda Barnes Foundation recommended a doctor nearby. He was current in nutrition as well as the specifics of CFS. He took my history and agreed to let me try T3, the active form of thyroid hormone. If your blood tests indicate that thyroid levels are high enough to meet accepted normal levels but your temperature is low - your body's problem may not be lack of the hormone but rather a problem using the hormone in general. I began on the graduated regimen of T3. You basically cycle up and then down until you capture a 98.6 average body temp. You can find details on Wilson's web page. I did several cycles and it did move my average daily temp from 98.0 to 98.3. I was certainly feeling better than I had in years!

My doctor put me on Cortef, a natural form of Cortisone, for three weeks. Short-term usage may allow the system to 'rest' and hopefully repair itself. This therapy is recommended in Dr. Jacob Teitelbaum's book, "From Fatigued to Fantastic." Dr. Teitelbaum's writing is a must for all CFS sufferers. Even if one doesn't follow his protocols to get better, having someone pinpoint and so accurately describe what you are feeling can be liberating.

The combination of T3 and cortisone made my days better, my depression less and led to the philosophy that I still follow today: "The straw that broke the camel's back."

I believe that we all face adversity and that we can usually handle one, two or three forces against us. It's when we have multiple attacks, whether it be stress, dehydration, toxins etc. that we eventually have too much, 'the Mantz Straw', and our body breaks down and we fall prey to illness and depression.

The cortisone and not struggling for a diagnosis may have helped my depression lift. My sleep improvements along with a better diet and a nice exercise regimen coupled with a smaller amount of ingested prescription medications, all may have allowed me to feel better, because I was not reaching the Mantz Straw on a daily basis.

I started a job as a head-hunter for an agency. I was now seeing three to four weeks in a row where I felt good. There was something right out in front of me that could get me over the edge but I just couldn't grasp what it was!

I stumbled upon an incredible site called Curezone. Dr. Richard Schulze aka Professor Cayenne and Dr. Christopher recommended cayenne. Believe me - cayenne in pill form is a learning experience. Take it with too little food and suffer the consequences. Sometimes getting out of the room quickly enough to double over is a chore when in an office setting! But I continued to take them and eventually eliminated my intake of T3 and cortisone. And I continued to feel good.

I learned that licorice might act as a food source of cortisone support so I added that.

I bought a juicer and started making fresh juice and began to make my own distilled water. I did Schulze's one week cleanses and later added the Epsom Salt Liver Cleanse. Headaches, which had been a major issue, were a thing of the past. The cleanses and the cayenne were my cure.

I learned about Apple Cider Vinegar. A tablespoon ten minutes before meals helps digestion. I got some at the health food store and began taking a tablespoon, a few drops of cayenne and a bit of distilled water before eating. I also stopped having liquids during meals. I have not had one symptom of IBS since that week! And - I no longer need Metamucil.

I decided to revisit my old allergist. I underwent the same skin scratch allergy tests that I had undergone some 20 years ago. They came back negative. I was no longer showing any signs of allergies at all. So, my allergies were cleared. My gut was good. My CFS continued to improve and Schulze and Curezone were my heroes!

I believe in the Straw theory and in eliminating prescription medications. Getting a good night's sleep and going to bed early. Stabilizing body temperature by exercising and through the use of cayenne. Only drinking distilled water and getting great nutrition through SuperFood and Udo's Choice. I always have a window cracked open, even in the dead of winter, to keep oxygen levels high inside my home.

I have chosen a few great friends over having many so-so friends. I am close with my family and have a fiancée who loves Schulze too! I no longer work in an office and I run an employment firm from home. I try to laugh as much as possible and I share my knowledge with whoever asks for it.

I don't rely on modern medicine for my cure but I do rely on it for diagnosis. I still have an amalgam filling in my mouth but would never fill a new cavity with anything but porcelain. One of the best books of all time is Dale Carnegie's, "How to Stop Worrying and Start Living." Everyone should read it.

My diet follows the same pattern. I am not a vegetarian or a vegan. I eat whatever I want supplemented by tons of fruits and vegetables. We find organic foods that do not contain any hydrolyzed or hydrogenated ingredients. We've eliminated milk from our diets and both have had about a 99% reduction in stuffy noses. If a recipe calls for milk, in it goes, but oatmeal is eaten sans milk or with Westsoy Unsweetened Soy Milk (plain or vanilla). We go through several bulbs of garlic per week. It kicks cholesterol and viruses in the butt. We use maple syrup instead of sugar to sweeten. We take two tablespoons of unsulphured blackstrap molasses every morning. One tablespoon provides 20% of your day's requirement of Calcium *and* Iron in a form that the body can actually use. Another great item is Green Tea.

I hope that you benefit from reading this story. Don't do everything at once. The ideas in the past few paragraphs were instituted over fifteen years. They are so easy to do if you do them one or two at a time. They work too. They are a blueprint for a long and healthy life. I have not felt weak in over three years as I write this!

OK, it is now 2008 and I haven't felt weak in over three years and counting since writing this. Yep, my CFS is dead, gone, cured!

Most useful aid to recovery - exercise and the stubbornness to lift weights even though at first I felt terrible for days after doing it. Cayenne. Drinking half your body weight in ounces of water per day without salt restrictions, and a regular sleeping pattern.

Recommended books
"From Fatigued to Fantastic" by D Jacob Teitelbaum
"How to Stop Worrying and Start Living" by Dale Carnegie
"Hypothyroidism, The Unsuspected Illness" by Broda Barnes

Most useful websites
www.lef.org
www.brodabarnes.org
www.wilsonssyndrome.com
www.drweil.com
http://return.to/organicherbs (Mountain Rose)
www.curezone.com
www.superfood.andmuchmore.com
www.dr.fuhrman.com
http://committed.to/bestdeals - for "Eat to Win" book by Dr Joel Furhman

Bob Mantz

Mandy's Story

Mickel Therapy was the turning point of my life

I can probably pinpoint the onset of my ME/CFS to over fifteen years ago. I wasn't aware I was suffering from ME at the time and so I continued to push myself, and undoubtedly made myself worse. I was in a very demanding job and under a lot of pressure at work. I was also juggling family life with my four year old and my partner, and around this time my mother was diagnosed with breast cancer. I got one virus after another, but blood tests showed that I was in perfect health. I tried reading books on fatigue and I bought expensive vitamins for energy and help with nerves. I also joined a gym as I decided I must need to get a few hours 'me' time, but little did I know that I was just making things worse for myself.

One day I physically couldn't get out of bed. When I finally managed to get to a chiropractor he asked if I'd been lifting anything heavy. I couldn't think of anything, so I was treated for sciatica. My back improved slightly after a few expensive sessions and I started back on life's roller coaster - work, family, gym, housework and social life. Then, after a night out in June/July 2004 with friends, I became violently ill and continued to be ill for a good three weeks. However, blood tests were again negative and so I thought I must have an intolerance to white wine.

By this stage my mother had been given the all clear and things had started to settle down at work and at home. I didn't get as stressed at work because my mother's illness had changed my priorities, and I decided, quite rightly, that there are more important things to worry about. But by November I was ill again. I was having a lot of time off work, but I couldn't explain how ill and extremely tired I was feeling, no matter how much sleep or rest I got. After a week off work I would go back ,even though I obviously wasn't well, and would explain my absence as 'flu'. After-all, if the blood tests said that I was OK, then I must be, and I should just pull myself together!

My birthday is at the end of November and my partner had arranged a lovely surprise weekend away in a hotel for the two of us, with a nice day of pampering just for me. On the morning we were due to travel I felt really ill, but I just couldn't explain *how* exactly, and I couldn't disappoint my partner after all the trouble he'd been to. I think that around when I knew something was seriously wrong with me. I remember washing up and smashing a plate and just breaking down crying. I thought I must be having some sort of a breakdown – and this was the start of my nerves being permanently on edge and being intolerant to noise of any sort. We had our weekend away. The massage I had was torture. The facial nice and relaxing. We had a lovely weekend - and then when we got back all I wanted to do was go to bed and sleep again.

However, I went to work the following week, much to my partner's disgust. Each night I'd have no energy and I literally made our meal, had a bath and went to bed. By the weekend I was sleeping around the clock again. I kept thinking there was something at home that was making me sleep as I seemed to be able to stay awake at work. In hindsight I think my body used up its total energy supplies at work and there was nothing left over for home.

I went to the doctor the following Monday and was seen by a locum GP who asked if I smoked. I didn't. So then he asked if I'd done my Christmas shopping. I foolishly thought he was trying to see how I'd exerted myself, but no, he thought I wanted time off to do my shopping. I was disgusted. He gave me diarrhoea powders and said I'd be bouncing after two days. I didn't waste any time arguing with him. I took the sachets for two days and made an appointment to see another doctor for a second opinion.

Luckily this doctor was more sympathetic and diagnosed chronic fatigue syndrome. On every visit afterwards I would ask about alternative therapies, medicines or help with looking after my four year old child - and then would cry when there was no solution.

I started reading up on ME and joined a support group. Unfortunately I found this very depressing as most of the members were long-term sufferers on disability benefits. However, I was able to get information from them about different alternative medicines.

After about a month off work and what I thought was a good rest, I re-started work in the New Year. However, I was ill again after only a week and back to square one. My condition worsened to the point where I was in bed five out of seven days, and the days on which I was up I could only manage to wash and dress and sit up to watch television. I felt like a zombie, watching the rest of the world go by. My mood was so low, and I was losing weight which I could ill afford. My hip and ankle joints were severely affected and I wasn't being paid from work any more and I worried about how we'd cope. My partner was coming in from work to look after me and our son, or if he was working away, then my elderly and disabled mother would stay to tend to me and Jack.

One day I read an article about anti-candida diets and in the first four to five weeks of trying this I saw an improvement. Brilliant I thought, I've cracked it! But five days later I was laid up again. By this point I was on Prozac, minimum dosage one a day.

The worst day of my life was a day that my mother was staying with me and my dad came down to take my son to school. It was only a five minute drive or ten minute walk – but I couldn't manage it. I'd only been out of bed for about an hour and was lying on the settee, yet each time I opened my eyes I got a blinding pain and it wouldn't stop. I went to lie in the bedroom in the dark in silence. My son was crying because he wanted his mummy to get him out of the bath and dress him – he was only four, bless him. My parents had to console him and were really worried about me. Eventually I must have fallen asleep and I woke up about four hours later.

Things between my partner and myself became strained because I just wanted to be left completely alone until I got better, but that wasn't happening. I couldn't bear any physical contact from him or my son. I couldn't even be bothered to make conversation. When my mother took two buses down to see me, I would practically slam the door in her face. I really did just want to be left alone in peace and quiet and didn't want anyone seeing me in such a state.

Prior to my illness I had been a happy, bubbly, sociable, confident and energetic person, but it seemed like that was part of another life. Before having my son I had a full time job *and* a part-time job. I had a hectic social life and went to the gym four or five times a week, and I still had energy to spare. Now I couldn't keep up my part-time job and home life without being ill, and getting out of bed was a bonus, and leaving the house an adventure.

We had to cancel our holiday to Portugal because I couldn't travel in a car at this stage without feeling sick. We were considering downsizing our three-bedroom cottage to a two-bedroom bungalow, as stairs were becoming a major problem. The guilt of my illness and being such a burden on all my loved ones and friends was so depressing. And it was so frustrating that on my good days I'd feel normal again - and then two days later be back to being an invalid!

One day, my partner's parents sent me a newspaper article on Mickel Therapy - and that was the turning point of my life. I found there was a therapist locally but the cost put me off at £80 per session. Was it just a scam? Was it making money out of peoples' misfortune? My partner persuaded me that I had nothing to lose and to give it a go, so I did. The first session was very painful for me, but I got through it and booked another one, and did the tasks

I'd been asked. After the first session and night's sleep I felt relaxed for the first time in months and years. My dreams and thoughts seemed to be opening up lots of old wounds, but they didn't seem to hurt any more.

After the second session I was doing great! I was getting out and about with my son to the park. I was making dinner for the family and driving. All normal things, but since my illness an absolute *joy* to be able to do them.

When I went for my third session and was told I didn't need any further sessions, that I was doing all I needed to do, I was *so* pleased with myself. And since then I've not looked back. I've had lots of things thrown at me since and I've coped with them better than I ever would have done in the past. I'm full of the joys of life and appreciation of my health, family and friends. Everything has been worthwhile. I sometimes get a little warning signal when I've overdone things, but now I take notice, and instead of pushing myself harder, I take a break.

I am also a lot more conscious of my diet. I've always eaten the daily five fruit and vegetables but am more aware of what I put into my body. I take my daily doses of vitamin C and also evening primrose oil and cod liver oil and I drink about four litres of water a day. I am determined that I will look after my body and health as I have discovered that it is too precious to risk losing again.

I started back at work about six weeks after my third session; two half-days a week, then three, then four and then back to five days. However, I make sure that I take a lunch break and I only do my set five hours, instead of doing seven hours without a break.

I've enjoy being out and about as much as possible with my son and partner. I also have regular nights out with my partner and friends. I don't think I'll ever be able to drink wine like I used to, but I seem to manage a few gin and tonics! Friends and family could not believe the difference in me in such a short space of time, nor could my GP. When asked what I put it down to, I say Mickel Therapy.

I am so grateful to my in-laws for sending me that article, because without it I think I'd still be bedridden and missing out on life.

Most useful aid to recovery - Mickel Therapy

Recommended website
www.mickeltherapy.com

Mandy's advice - good nutrition helps. I try to avoid sugar, yeast and alcohol and I've cut out caffeine completely. Try to play and rest twice as much as you work and you'll reap the benefits!

Mandy Robson

Tom's Story

ME – an illness not for children

Tom was born in 1991. As a baby he had many ear infections, until grommets were fitted. He didn't have a big appetite and he didn't sleep well, in fact, Tom was nearly three years old before he started sleeping through the night, and by this time, his sister had arrived. Other than this Tom was a normal healthy boy.

At the age of five Tom started getting hay fever and each year thereafter it got worse. He did, however, take up football and joined a local boy's team and he would attend practice and play a game every week during the football season.

In January 2001 when Tom was nine, he contracted Glandular Fever. He was very poorly and missed over half of year five in Primary School. Also, during the summer, Tom's hay fever was so bad that it brought on an asthma attack and he was put on a nebuliser and steroids. This, on top of his glandular fever symptoms, meant that Tom was again very ill. Unfortunately he had to give up his football, and though some of the boys kept in contact for a short time, as Tom became more ill, they stopped calling.

Due entirely to his strength of character Tom was able to go back to school for Year six but he couldn't do any sport and still had days off with chronic tiredness, sore throats and joint pain. Luckily he is a very bright boy and did his Year six SATS exams with average grades in Science and Maths and above average in English. We couldn't have asked for more considering the amount of education he had missed.

We all decided that we should visit the two high schools which Tom could attend.

The first school provided transport from home and it was also where all Tom's school friends would be going. The second school meant I would have to drive him, but it did have a good reputation. After visiting both schools Tom decided that he would prefer to go to the second school, and we agreed with him. We thought it was a very brave move of his, as it meant he would start secondary school with no friends and he would have to make new friends.

In September 2002, at eleven years old, Tom began at the new high school. Unfortunately though, by the October half-term we could see that Tom was looking and feeling ill, and a visit to the doctor proved fruitless as he just said it was the after- effects of glandular fever. The three hours sport Tom was doing every week at school began to take its toll and by December 2002 his lack of appetite was worrying us very much and he looked constantly tired. We decided to see the doctor again but I got the same response as before. However, this time though he did do a blood test; but of course it came back negative and the doctor's words were "there is nothing wrong with him". During the Christmas holiday Tom slept for twelve to fourteen hours a day and Christmas was a non-event for all of us.

Tom did manage to go back to school in January but his health deteriorated so fast that within three weeks he could hardly get out of bed. He was hardly eating and sometimes didn't even know what day it was. One day I managed to get him dressed and practically carried him in to see our GP, and the reaction I got was appalling. His comments were, and I quote "he does look ill, but I do not know what is wrong with him. He is just lazy and doesn't want to go to school!" At this we left the surgery, with me in tears and Tom dazed, not really knowing what was going on.

At this point as a family we realised we were on our own. Our desperation was coming to a head when my husband saw an article in the Sunday Times about how Lady Clare Kerr, the daughter of Michael Ancram the MP, had received treatment from the Breakspear Hospital for ME and how, after years of illness, she was now leading a normal life. Was this the light at the end of our tunnel?

The next day I telephoned the Breakspear and spoke to a senior doctor there. After explaining Tom's illness and that he was only eleven years old, she very kindly made room in her busy schedule to see him straight away, despite the fact that they had a waiting list. The hospital sent me a questionnaire asking lots of questions about Tom's health which I had to complete and take with me to the appointment. The questionnaire confirmed the fact that Tom was borderline acute illness.

The appointment was in February 2003. After the first consultation the doctor confirmed that Tom was ill with ME/Chronic Fatigue Syndrome. At last we had confirmation that Tom was ill. At last someone believed Tom and believed us! Whilst we had a cup of coffee in the waiting room a nurse worked out Tom's treatment regime, together with the costs. The cost of the treatment was more expensive than we had expected but we had to give it a try as our son was wasting away in front of our eyes. We had to try it whatever the cost. After discussions we agreed that we would go ahead with the treatment but if we saw no signs of improvement after two or three months we would re-evaluate our decision. We were in BUPA at the time but they said Tom's illness was not covered.

We approached our local Primary Care Trust who, to say the least, treated us very badly – but that is another story. Needless to say they said Tom would get better in time and they would not fund what they considered to be "fringe" treatment. They also implied that the treatment was dangerous. The PCT did arrange for Tom to see a specialist doctor but we felt this meeting was to vet us as parents, not in fact to help Tom. What a waste of time and Tom's energy.

Tom visited the Breakspear Hospital at the beginning of March 2003 and his treatment started with injections to ascertain what his allergies were. Then the hospital made up vaccines for food allergies and chemical allergies. Tom would have to have one injection of each every day. He was also given vitamin B12. All of this was carried out in one day and we all returned home exhausted. As well as the vaccine, Tom was given a course of vitamins, which totalled twenty-seven tablets per day. These were, of course, introduced gradually. It all soon became a daily routine, but not a pleasant one. I hated giving him the injections and he hated having them. Tom would put a towel covered ice block on his arm to freeze the skin a little so he did not feel the needles as badly. We split his tablets during the day but Tom still didn't like taking them.

After just one week of treatment Tom was eating better than he had for some months. Within four weeks a lot of his symptoms had eased considerably. Within three months a lot of the symptoms had totally subsided and he was able to start thinking about going back to school. The difference in him was remarkable! He was putting on weight and he was growing in height, which we had noticed had stopped since being diagnosed with glandular fever. In fact his sister was almost as tall as him and almost as heavy. As time went on the recovery time did slow down and we still did have times of Tom being very tired but overall he was still improving.

In June 2003 Tom started back to school doing just a couple of hours a day. We continued on this regime and gradually Tom attended more hours each week. We were so relieved at how much better he was looking until he had a very bad asthma attack and he was admitted to hospital. He was on a nebuliser for twenty-four hours and given steroids. I explained to the nurses that Tom was having treatment for ME and they confirmed that they were happy for him to take his medication whilst in the hospital if we wanted him to. However, Tom was very ill and I thought he was going through enough, so the treatment stopped for three days until he returned home.

By Christmas 2003 Tom felt able to cope without the vaccine so we stopped the injections, but he still took the vitamins.

Over the following months Tom improved at a steady pace and by year nine he was only missing the odd day off school. He took up skateboarding and most Saturdays would meet his friends at the skate park. It was great to see him enjoying life! The cheekiness of a teenager had arrived - more signs that he was recovering.

Tom started year ten as a healthy fourteen year old. He went off skateboarding and took up golf - a lot of walking! He now plays eighteen holes of golf most Fridays and sometimes does nine holes in the week or goes to the Driving Range. He also likes to watch car racing and visit car exhibitions with his Dad. Recently he did two weeks work experience at a local car manufacturer, getting up at 6.00 am every morning and returning home at 4.00 pm. He unfortunately caught a cold the second week but still managed to go to work. He can't wait to start work properly.

We are so proud of the way Tom handled his illness and would also like to say how considerate and thoughtful his sister was throughout all of Tom's illness - she was brilliant.

Whilst the Breakspear wouldn't suit everyone, we feel that without this hospital Tom wouldn't be as fit and healthy again as he is now.

Most useful aid to recovery - The Breakspear Hospital, UK

Recommended website - www.breakspearhospitaltrust.org.uk

Kim's advice - When Tom was feeling particularly down we would always revert back to the old saying "there is always someone worse off than you" and this helped to keep us all going.

Kim Bickley (Tom's mother)

Patricia's Story

An exercise programme where you move no more than an inch

It was a *nightmare!* Does that sound dramatic or neurotic or both? Well, lucky you if it does. You obviously haven't got, have never had, or never lived with anyone, suffering with myalgic encephalomyelitis/ chronic fatigue syndrome.

Commonly known as ME, this abominable scourge on young and old alike picked on little old me as its hostess for a good ten years. Don't panic fellow sufferers, that does not mean that your visit by this nightmare will be anywhere near as long. Some have much milder symptoms and some recover within months.

I tried hard not to accommodate my unwelcome, twenty-four hour, nightmare visitor. Now living alone, with my two sons with homes and families of their own, I was enjoying my work. Working thirty hours at my day job and about twenty more at night as a barmaid, what time had I got for feeling so tired and unwell? They do say that about ME sufferers don't they? We're always on the go, giving 110% at whatever we do.

So when did this nightmare begin? I pin it down to a rough bout of flu and sore throat, both of which never seemed to completely leave me. The day job had also become extremely stressful under new management but I had always thrived on adrenaline so got on with it like the rest of my colleagues. I began having long sleepless nights. I'd get up mornings with my body desperately longing to lie in bed all day, but my spirit as always, told me to get up and get to work. However, some days I just couldn't make it.

How *was* I feeling exactly? Do I really have to tell you out there? I'm sure you could write a book yourself. Apart from the loss of sleep and the bad dreams when I did manage to sleep, I had aches and pains all over my body. Coupled with the feeling of extreme fatigue that seemed to surpass mere tiredness, walking and standing was difficult and sitting not much better. Lying flat out seemed to ease things, but you can't do that in the middle of the electricity board showroom floor in front of customers.

There was something that I did manage in front of customers though – losing my memory. Years of experience meant I could 'wing' the intricacies of the workings of the various washing machines or cookers as I helped Mr or Mrs Bloggs to choose a new appliance. But when it came to taking their details, I failed miserably. Sitting in front of the computer I would inquire "Your name and address please?", "Mrs. Joe Bloggs, 22 Acacia Avenue, Midtown, Westside, Wombledon, SY99 8ZZ." Would be something like their answer.

My answer would be something like, "Is that Blogg or Bloggs with an S?" That would be my way of trying to bide some time while I racked my brain to remember what else they had said. Or "Can you say that again dear? I'm sure I've got earwax." It became so bad that customers would give me worried looks, wondering if I was fit to work out their hire purchase agreement properly. I felt a proper 'Charlie'. My memory had been almost photographic. I could read a page from a book and practically recite it word for word. Now I couldn't even hear an address and write it down as it was being spoken!

A frightening episode happened one day when a good friend whom I had known for years, was taking me out in the car. He was telling me the name of another friend's new baby, that it was the same as his. I looked at him and thought, 'What *is* your name?' It was one of the most frightening times of the whole illness. It wasn't a momentary lapse as we all have, it took me about ten minutes to discover his name. I did it by thinking of how I could get him to say it himself. I remembered he had more than one name, so asked him innocently, "Which one of your names did you say they'd called him?" Even when I heard the name, my brain wouldn't immediately relate it to the person sitting by my side.

Total fatigue enveloped my whole being and I ached as though I'd been run over by the bus I now took to and from work, instead of the ten minute walk. After work, the bus would drop me a hundred yards from home. No, surely it was ten miles? I willed myself to put one foot in front of the other. Oh the joy of reaching that front door to my block of flats. Oh the despair as I faced the two flights of stairs to number eleven. I christened them my own personal Mount Everest. "Please don't let anyone come out and see me" would be my one thought as I undertook that first flight, one painful step at a time. Then I would turn the corner and lean on the banister, making my way to the next thirteen steps, where I would often as not have to sit for several minutes before I ascended on all fours. There were times I would reach the top landing and lie on the floor before I could make the final eight-foot stretch to my front door. Once inside I often lay on the hall floor for up to ten or more minutes before I regained enough energy to get up and sprawl on the bed or settee. Retelling it now I can hardly believe it was that bad, but trust me folks, it was.

My good friend and neighbour Herbie knocked on my door one day, holding a small dining chair. "I got this from a car boot" he beamed "I'm going to put it at the bottom of our stairs so you can rest on it between flights." I could have cried at his thoughtfulness. The next day I crawled home as usual. The thought of the chair waiting for me egged me up that first hurdle. "Isn't this great?" piped up dear old Mrs Haynes. "Herbie has put a chair out. I'm going to enjoy sitting here watching the world go by." She looked me up and down like a farmer assessing a horse for the knackers yard. "Whatever's the matter with you? You look dreadful." I wanted to cry, "Get off that ruddy chair, it was meant for me!" But she was so delighted, bless her. Over the years, I would sit on the stairs as usual until I got my breath back while she continued to tell me how ill I looked, but she never rendered up the chair. Herbie did provide a second seat, but Mrs Haynes's friend from the flat opposite joined her in her daily vigil. It gave some of us great pleasure to see the two old dears putting the world to rights over their substitute for a garden fence, but sadly, there wasn't room for *three* seats.

One day an old friend telephoned. I remember her saying, "Are you OK Pat? No you're not. Don't move. I'll be there in ten minutes." I was still on the floor in the hall when she arrived. I was petrified and in tears. She thought I was having a breakdown and in a way, I suppose I was. Bless you my namesake friend for making me go to the doctor. I insisted on the last appointment of the day, knowing that I would be in pieces from the effort of getting there and afraid of making a fool of myself in front of other patients. Thankfully, I saw a recently new doctor to our practice and he was absolutely wonderful. I agreed to the antidepressant amitriptyline, to help me sleep, and he gave me a sick note for a month off work. Joy of joys. A whole month to rest and get better. Who was I kidding? It continued to become much worse in spite of some drug induced, welcome sleep.

Discovering that the pains in my body were greatly eased by a good long hot soak, some days I would have two, three, or even four long baths. Friends and family were amused that I would take the phone in the bathroom. They never knew how many hours I spent in that tub. In fact, they never knew a lot about the whole process really.

We have never been a family who visits every week. How I loved and hated their visits when they came. They never knew how hard it was trying to take in what they said. They were unaware of the pain of just sitting upright in the chair, or of me, loving them so very much, yet wishing they would go, because I felt as though my whole being was being painfully abused by the trauma of my body and brain trying to behave normally. I couldn't make conversation. I winced at the noise of theirs.

All the time I was frightened at what was happening to me. What was wrong with me? I even developed an allergy/intolerance to paint and chemical fumes and certain perfumes and deodorants.

Well, it's all been doom and gloom about my nightmare so far, but how did I get back on track?

When things got bad, and even badder, when the relapses occurred, yet again, when I felt that no one understood or even cared, I just gritted my teeth and very firmly reminded myself of one of my late mother's old sayings; "Don't let the b.....s get you down girl!" Sometimes I wouldn't succeed, but most times it was sheer determination that I *would* get well, that I *would not* be beaten that kept me going. What a gift has been my ability to laugh at my misfortunes, although I know some think I am flippant. They have no idea! My tears are always my personal possession.

Going to bed at night, I refused to dwell on the day's negativity. I stopped beating myself up for the things I hadn't or couldn't do. Instead, I went over the positive things I had achieved that day. Maybe just the fact that I had prepared and cooked a proper meal; that I'd managed to watch the whole half hour of Coronation Street on television, or that I had climbed those stairs on two paws, not four. On bad days I counted the good days, reminding myself that they *were* happening and would one day overtake the bad.

I listened to my instincts. In the beginning, when I hadn't the energy to turn over in bed, when lifting my hand to scratch my head took every ounce of strength, I knew instinctively that being so immobile could lead to being permanently unable to get up out of my bed. It frightened me so much that I knew I had to fight this nightmare invasion of my mind and body. The strange thing was it was one of the symptoms of that nightmare that put me on the track to some self-help. Lying in bed, I not only had aches and pains, but I had what I can only describe as a creepy crawly sensation in my whole being. Something like 'fidgety legs' but all over. I wanted to move, to shake myself to rid myself of this awful sensation, but even wriggling my toes was exhausting. I couldn't get to sleep because of it, I couldn't get comfortable to rest and it drove me to distraction. So I devised a method of what I came to call my 'Fidget' exercises to try to help me relax.

Initially it was difficult to carry out because just wriggling my toes would exhaust me. However, I quickly realized that what I was trying to do would help me keep the oxygen and circulation going in my limbs. I lay in bed and thought of how I could extend these 'fidgets' to the whole of my body - just small movements of wriggling and flexing toes, arms and legs. And breathing exercises to get the oxygen into my blood. It could all be done lying on my back in bed. It was many months before I could go from toe to top in one session, but I made sure I did something every evening. One thing it succeeded in was tiring me out enough to get some sleep. I can't describe how hard it was to persevere, but instinct told me to do so. Can you believe an exercise program where you moved nothing more than an inch? (See below).

Once I could eat properly, I made sure it was sensibly. Very early on I exchanged my intolerance for tea, coffee and alcohol for Earl Grey, hot chocolate and water. I popped the vitamins and evening primrose, tried the gingko biloba, glucosamine and anything else that took my fancy, that I could afford. Did they help? Sometimes I think they did, sometimes I was unsure. Ginkgo and evening primrose seemed worth it. Eventually, I weaned myself off the amitriptyline in the hope that the fog would lift and I could find my old self again. I'm not advocating that you follow that particular course without your doctor's knowledge and supervision.

Suffering for years with what was diagnosed as arthritis in my neck, a friend sung the praises of her magnetic bracelets. I was sceptical but she convinced me it was worth a go. Not being a bracelet person, I bought a watch instead, and swore to wear it each day for at least three months. It kept excellent time. Unfortunately, after two years I still had the pain in the neck! *But,* about six weeks after purchasing it I threw the pillow on the settee and settled down for my usual afternoon kip to recharge the old battery. Five minutes later it dawned on me that I wasn't in the least bit tired. Now come on! Afternoon bye byes had become as necessary to my life as breathing in and out. Sitting up, bewildered, I realized my fuzzy head was no longer fuzzy. What other way can I describe it? My brain felt light and airy as though it had had a spring-clean. Yes, that does sound daft but I am trying hard to explain it. I was over the moon, yet very puzzled. The next day I still felt the improvement – could it be the magnetic bracelet on my watch? Who knows, but I certainly did not imagine the feeling of well-being and have since heard of other ME sufferers who have had good results with magnets.

Spending time alone was boring, so I visited elderly ladies in the sheltered complex next door. In past bad times I had learned that helping others less fortunate would put my own troubles into perspective. It has also always given me great joy. They believed I was being benevolent towards them and were extremely grateful for my company. Not so, I loved them dearly and they made my life worth living. They taught me about life and how precious it is.

My son gave me my first computer and slowly I began writing again. I did the neighbourhood news for the local rag. Nothing major, but it gave me a sense of achievement. I had a few poems published in anthologies. So, you can see that improvements were being made. These activities were only possible when they *were* possible if you see what I mean. Good days were used to the full, although the price had to be paid. Oh how I loved those good days. Not just for what I achieved during them, but because they were the sunlight on the horizon, the brilliance at the end of the tunnel, the pleasant dream that would one day completely annihilate my long, drawn-out nightmare.

I dug out my oils and did a little painting. I took up decoupage. I did anything that was positive for my ego. Gradually I was able to achieve good mornings *most* days, although I needed an afternoon rest. I had long given up on a social life as friends had moved on and anyway, the ME was too unreliable. I feared making plans and promises that I may have to break. Early nights gave me good mornings, sometimes whole good days. Staying home nights was worth the price. Life was gradually creeping back.

By 2000, I had made vast improvement, although I still had to rest most days, as well as conserve some energy for future plans. But the nightmare wasn't so scary anymore. I so wanted to get back to work and when I began having some good days I would browse the situations vacant column in the local paper. Maybe, just maybe, there would be something *very* part-time that I could accomplish? Perhaps even some work at home? Then I reasoned that what employer would put up with someone who didn't turn in on certain days every week because the nightmare was visiting? NO. I wasn't going to let that stop me. So, on good mornings I began to get up as *though* I had already got work. I showered, dressed, and would sit writing at my computer for a set period of time - just to see how long a day I could manage and how many days in a row it would last. Or, I would visit my old ladies and stay a certain length of time. I tried to pace myself to test my reliability as a future employee. Sometimes I thought I did quite well and other times I got more than a little depressed as I realized I wasn't yet ready.

There was one wonderfully up-lifting experience during my search for the perfect employment. I spotted a job that I had often thought I would love to tackle. This company was looking for a coach courier; someone to look after holidaymakers in this country and on the continent. Being a 'people person' this was just up my street! However, I hadn't applied for a job since 1978 and here it was the year 2000 and you were expected to have a curriculum vitae. Whatever that was! It took me a while, but I wrote a great one. Before the reply landed on my doorstep I was feeling pretty fatigued, but the interview was three weeks away so hopefully I could conserve energy and plan a good day for it. Yes I did say interview, my first interview for twenty years. I was elated and petrified. The day arrived and I could have felt a lot better, but a little blusher and lipstick are wonderful inventions.

It was a group interview! That threw me. Listening to the job requirements and trying hard to accommodate the hubbub of voices made me realize that I wouldn't be able to commit to my dream job. I didn't wait to see if I'd be successful, I told them I didn't want it on my way out, explaining my reasons with a deep apology. Did I despair? I did not! My first application in all those years and I was one of ten short-listed out of a hundred and twelve. What's more, they led me to believe that I would have stood a good chance of getting it. I felt pretty good about that. I'd done it once, so I could do it again.

As it happened, I took up voluntary work and in 2001 when I reached sixty I decided to manage on my pension. However, I'm out all day Monday, Tuesday and Wednesday mornings, am chairperson of a social club, edit a sixteen page newsletter for a voluntary organisation, am trying to write a novel and have just begun painting again.

Gradually my days brightened and my fatigue lessened. Some of the things I've mentioned helped, but I believe the CFS just ran its course and I now get on with my life. It's wonderful to be able to make plans, go on holiday, walk without sinking to the floor and to once again enjoy a glass of wine. I'm even back on the coffee, though it is only cappuccino, and I have become a convert to Earl Grey tea.

Very occasionally, the thought of what I endured makes me angry. However, it has taught me compassion and tolerance for the plight of others. It has taught me not to judge. I hope it has made me a better person - but it was one hell of a learning curve! I still mourn those years of my life, spent lost in the nightmare of ME. I must remember to appreciate the years to come. The important thing is that I have survived *my* nightmare and you *will* survive yours!

Most useful aid to recovery - magnetic watch. Patience.

Recommended website - www.worldofmagnets.co.uk

Patricia's advice - it's so easy now for me to say don't despair, but please try not to. Each day that passes may seem very hard, but remember, it's *one day nearer to recovery*. Begin by doing one positive thing each day and gloating on it before you go to bed.

Don't be like me and not ask for help. It will keep your friends and family around you. Remember to explain that you do love and appreciate them, even though it may seem as though you can't cope with their company. Halfway through my ordeal I had a new neighbour who did untold good for me - thank you Hazel for being a true friend, then and now. Laugh at yourself. Listen to happy music, watch comedy videos, find something to do that will give you some sense of worth. Write a poem, draw, paint, knit, do jigsaws or whatever tiny thing gives you some pleasure. Get a cat, a goldfish or a canary. Something to watch, to cuddle, (don't cuddle the goldfish!) something to care for.

Whenever possible, don't forget to FIDGET and wriggle those toes and fingers and flex those arms and legs. The smallest movements are better than nothing at all. Join your local ME/CFS society and get informed! Membership will also provide you with listening ears from those who truly do know what you are going through, and there are usually some social get-togethers to make new friends.

Patricia Franklin

Max's Story

One man's inner experience and cure

Dear friend, relative, or person with CFS ...my name is Max Rivers. I contracted CFS in January 1994 and then was cured two days after taking Hanna Kroeger's homeopathic BE. Kit. (BE stands for Bar Epstein - being German, Hanna often reversed words). I feel a deep responsibility to share my experience about this wonderful remedy with other people with CFS. As a computer programmer and not a homeopath, all I can really do is pass on my own personal experience.

For some reason, having no arms wasn't it, really, although looking back it's hard to believe that that part of the hallucination didn't startle me. It wasn't even being required by the Nazis to crawl around on our bellies, never standing up, or doing anything not allowed. It was the incredible complacency of the others. No one else seemed to care that we were in a concentration camp on the island of Jamaica, at the hands of a Nazi Commandant. Well I did. And I secretly plotted to get away by sea. I didn't care if I got caught and killed. I wasn't going to live the rest of my life as a prisoner.

As it turns out, of course, I didn't have to, because four days later the fever broke and I found myself tangled up in soaking sheets, stale with four day old sweat, but safe in my bedroom. And wiped out.

A few days later, when my energy didn't return, I thought it was odd. A month later when I still felt exactly as I had the day my fever broke, I realized that I was really sick. So I gathered myself up, like so many broken pieces of a puzzle, like too many books to carry at once and drove to the doctor's. Within a few minutes he had his diagnosis - chronic fatigue syndrome. I had CFS.

Being diagnosed with chronic fatigue is like moving into a hospice. One minute you are too tired for words and the next your whole life is changed by three words. Oh, it isn't fatal, but it is 'incurable'. Or at least the doctors don't have a treatment for it yet. On my way out of the doctor's office I grew heavier with each step I took. No one knows how to stop this. It could just go on and on.

People look at you differently, with sad eyes, but fearful and a little frantic. I saw them looking in at me but I was too tired to really care. And I was too scared. I never really let myself feel just how scared I was. I let the fog of CFS protect me from the harsh reality of CFS. I knew in some vague way that if I ever actually looked the disease right in the face I would shatter into pieces like a glass dropped from a great height onto a hard, white tile floor - pieces of me flying off under things never to be returned. So instead I stayed vague about it. Calm and soft-edged and fuzzy.

That was alright for interacting with the world, but on a personal, day to day level, my body just plain hurt. It ached, like staying up and staying up and staying up, till you just can't keep your eyes open and then about an hour after you finally fall asleep the alarm goes off and you have to get up to drive across country - and your head is full of cotton and your arms are heavy as lead and your feet are too far away to feel and light knives through your eyes and your body aches like the color red - except that you just had twelve hours sleep and it still feels just like that. And if you rest you feel worse. Groggy and cob webs that you shake off with a huge effort of will, which only gets you back to aching like the color red and knives in your eyes.

At first it seems to everyone and even you that all you need is an effort of will to get above it, but like quicksand, that is just what it wants you to think.

You see, CFS has a Nazi Commandant that doesn't want to punish you, but what can he do? He has to make an example of you and so he punishes you for your every effort, with a flu-like illness that comes on like lightning, fever and chills and headache and bone ache for two or three days, for just the effort of will to disobey him. And the rules change as time goes by, getting stricter and stricter until you aren't allowed to do anything at all, and still there are violations that get punished and it feels like the ceiling gets lower and lower until if you stand up tall, that is a violation, and down you go.

I became like one of those outdoor thermometers with some blood red substance which was sitting down there at the bottom, just below my belly, and it was my energy. And I could raise it up, pulling at the liquid with the fingers of my will, raising it up like trying to lift a rock with just your eyes, straining up and up until the blood red liquid would stain the white, papery, dry place that was my mind, soaking it up with a thirst that drained my last efforts after such a short time. At first all I could manage was half an hour of not quite clear headedness, but after a few short months it was more like half a minute before the Commandant would come and pull me off the fence and drag me back to be punished.

And I would lie there, sick and sweating, confused inside of a forgetfulness that is so complete that after a while all it is about is forgetting. But the saddest part was when my mind began to go. It's funny that the feeling was just numbing sadness, but that's what it was. My doctor even said that it was just part of the disease, that there would likely be some Alzheimer's-like forgetting, and that it would go away when the disease did. But he didn't mention the sadness of being without my mind for months and months and months.

And everything else is just out of reach: people and work and joy and interest. Books I can't read anymore because my eyes don't focus without effort and the Commandant won't allow that. So I lie there under water trying to rest through all the exhaustion, when a huge steel bell sounds piercing and sudden in one of my ears, more and more frequently, but my arms are too heavy to raise them to cup away the sound, which doesn't matter anyway, because the sound is inside my head. It is my exhaustion ringing like a bell every time I go too far.

And every now and again, just to exercise my sense of irony, I get up and walk around. It isn't that you're dizzy, it is just that you are now past the point where the effort to balance can be ignored. Once as I walked down the hall, one hand on the wall to make it easier, my lover came around the corner yelling at me that I am not making love with her frequently enough anymore - and at first it seems so ludicrous, like raging at me for not enunciating my Japanese, when I don't even speak Japanese, that I am relieved and grateful to her for so great a departure from the hell I have been rotting in - until a few weeks later when she takes a lover who 'satisfies her needs' and I realize that I am not to be spared anything that this disease has to offer and I realize that I would probably be devastated, if there was any more room for devastation, which there wasn't.

At this point it is five or six months. Work isn't even remotely possible, my lover has left, friends are all freaked, family is worried and require constant soothing, so basically it is me, alone with the Commandant.

This is not like me, facilitator of men's support groups for fifteen years now, so as soon as I hear about a CFS support group at Holyoke Hospital, even though it is farther than I have ventured out in months, I rest for days ahead of time and make the forty mile trip. What I find there horrifies me. Men and women my age, with stories just like mine, type "A" baby boomers, but most of them are six or seven years into this disease thing - that long or longer since they worked or played and since their lovers left. That long or longer since they gave up. A room full of waiting. Only the Commandant seems pleased. Everyone else seemed devolved. Some, the lucky ones, had become snails, the hard shell of doom wrapped around them like blankets; their soft, out of focus faces peaking out radiating weakness. The worst cases had become cocoons. CFS had wrapped itself around them and wrapped and wrapped and now they waited patiently, as their bodies softened and lost definition, changing into something else, shrouded in disease and given over to the process, wherever it may take them.

As I walked outside into the parking lot, my humanity stood before me like a little girl, wide-eyed as the crowd of us were marched off to the gas chamber. Her eyes asked the silent question, "What about me?" And as her mother, marching right along side of her to the same destiny, what was I supposed to answer? But an answer was required. This child before me was my last connection to being human. I was about to be dragged into the insect world, snail or caterpillar, it didn't matter. I was days away from the end of my life as a human. And there didn't seem to be anything I could do about it. I have always been a hopeful person. When I got home, I saw my hope waiting for me on the kitchen table. It was like some gadget that I knew I owned, but I couldn't remember how to work. Or maybe it just needed batteries. I hadn't lost my hope. I just didn't know how to work it anymore.

A few days later found me at the retreat center at the top of Mt. Temenos near my home in western Massachusetts. There were fifteen of us, all men. We were there to do a sweat lodge - an intense Native American ritual for making contact with the source of your own spirit. I was going to ask that spirit what to do next. I needed guidance. From someone besides the Commandant.

The men were great (men are great, aren't they!). They brought me my meals and built the lodge without me. They let me sleep in the main building and doze off any time I needed to. I was terrified about the lodge. They are very demanding, physically, and I suspected that the Commandant would torture me right well when I returned. But I noticed that he was not present on the mountain and I was determined to ask my question, if not for my own pain, then for that little girl's.

Inside the lodge, as the air heated past endurance, my skin began to vibrate with virus. Screaming that couldn't be heard was crawling over and under my skin, but I was used to that; the unusual part of the experience was deeper inside. I felt calm in there and healed. And that was the first message from the spirit of the lodge. The core of me was not affected by the disease. There was a rich, healthy core of meat that was my centre, that was untouched and unchanged. My humanity sighed a collective sigh and settled back into my core. A human ever more.

"What can I do to stop this train from running me over?" I asked. "What is it that you want me to know, what must I learn, look at, see, say, understand? I will do whatever it takes. I commit to you and to me and to this process fully. I commit to my soul."

This was not the first time that this was required of me. Fourteen years ago when I turned thirty my soul announced that it had a feminine side and so I rented the bridal suite at a hotel, and bought myself jewelry and the most expensive dinners on the menu. I wined and dined my female, as if she were another lover and I returned a changed man, with a new name, Max Rivers. And again on my fortieth, after a week of silence, on the moment of my birth, 2:20pm, I was told to learn to dance. I had never danced in my life, and that Friday and every Friday for two years I went to Dance Friday and I learned to dance and that I had a body and a spirit. So the spirit which spoke to me through the hardship of the lodge knew that all it had to do was ask and I would meet the answer.

And the message came. A name. "Hanna."

After the lodge I was lying naked on the earth. The men ran to the pond and dunked themselves in the icy water, screaming. And then they came back with buckets of water, and dowsed me as I lay in the, now, mud.

Suddenly I knew what it meant. A woman who ran a health food store in Boulder Colorado where I had lived twenty years ago, had healed me a few times when I had minor ailments the doctors couldn't figure out. I was to go to Boulder again.

The next weekend I was at a gathering of friends and a woman I barely knew came up to me and angrily shouted at me, "I want you to know I don't believe in these things!" "What things?" I asked. "Every time I look at you I see mountains in the background. What is that?" "I am going to Colorado to be healed," I whispered. "Well go already," she shouted. "I don't believe in these things. So go already!"

So the next day I bought a one-way ticket to Denver. I didn't even ask about the fares coming back. I would handle that when I got better. My soul likes one-way tickets. It shows commitment. I also didn't call Hanna. She had been a little old lady twenty years ago and I was afraid she might be dead and gone. But I knew better than to call. I had to go and find out. And I didn't call Hanna for twenty-one days after I got there. The CFS specialist I had gone to see put me on a twenty-one day supported fast and so I only drank powdered rice protein and water for twenty-one days. And I read "Care of the Soul." And I prepared myself for getting well.

It was a fascinating time for me, a type "A" person, to just fast for nearly a month and not do anything. I couldn't work or even think really and I could only read about a paragraph at a time and the rest of the time I just sat and watched the mountains and felt my body. Twice a week I went to a 'Course in Miracles' classes and once a week I did Tai Chi and that was it. The Commandant got bored and turned his attention elsewhere.

Before I left Shutesbury I had a healing session with a Reiki healer. She told me that 'virus' was the plural of 'Viron', the individual entities that make up an illness; that they weren't malevolent; they were just a particular kind of being that liked a particular kind of habitat and that I had become the perfect summer cottage for a colony of CFS virons.

I thought a lot about that. In truth I had vacated my body a lot this lifetime. The time I didn't spend in my mind I was in spirit. My body was a vessel to me, like a Chevy Van. I felt very clearly that I had left that big sliding door on the side of the van open and had walked away for so long that the virons had just moved in. And when I came back one day, there was no room left for me. I was the victim of an accidental sublet.

On the evening of the twenty-first day of the fast I found a scrap of paper that someone had given me with a number they'd had for Hanna several years ago. I called it and found out that Hanna had a retreat center about five blocks from where I was staying and that she was teaching a five day self-healing workshop starting that night, in about two hours. So I packed one bag of clothes and a friend drove me over to the 'Peaceful Meadow's Retreat Center'. Just as we drove up Hanna was walking out the front door towards us. She looked exactly the same, a little over four feet tall with the thickest German accent I've ever heard. She looked up at me as I got out of the car and cackled, "What's the matter with you?" "I have Chronic Fatigue," I said to her, dejectedly. "Chronic Fatigue?" she screeched, "Oh that's no problem. Two days." And she grabbed my hand in hers and dragged me, astonished and relieved beyond words, into the chapel, where she went behind a curtain and came out with a white box labeled 'B. E. Kit'. She put the box into my left hand, and reached into her apron and pulled out the same pendulum she'd used so many years ago, when last I'd gone to see her. She held it over the box in my hand and it swung wildly. "See!" she screamed, "Two days. No problem. Now get yourself settled because dinner is in a little vile and zen ve get started." And she hobbled off quickly, just like some character in Alice in Wonderland.

Up in my room, I opened the box. It contained a bottle of homeopathic liquid and two jars of green, herbal pills and a sheet which said to take fifteen drops and two pills from each bottle with each meal for two weeks. I took my first dose right then and went down to dinner. Classes went far into the night and all day the next day, with me taking a dose with each meal. During one class, I got very fatigued and went to the back of the room to lie down. Hanna, who was lecturing at the time, stopped and ran back towards me. "I don't like this, this is not good," she said to the class, as if still part of her lecture. She had me sit up and ran her pendulum over different parts of my body. "See?" she said (though none of us could see anything expect her pendulum swaying this way and that) the energy goes out here," she said holding the swinging pendulum in front of my face, "but does not come in here"; she held it behind my head and I gathered that it stopped moving. She 'tutted' like a sad grandmother and held my head in her hands and prayed to Jesus to help me. "There." she said with finality, as if something obvious had just taken place. "Now it is okay." And she went back to her lecture. I sat up, still feeling exactly as exhausted as I had a moment ago, but somehow buoyed up by her faith. Had something happened? I shushed my mind into quietness and chose Hanna's confidence over my fear. For the time being.

That night, during the evening lecture, one of her advanced students was teaching the class and Hanna sat off to the side, watching. Suddenly she stood up and walked right in front of the lecturer and grabbed my hands in hers and said," So. You have had the courage to look your truth in the face. And so you will be healed. Yah." The two women students on either side of me burst into tears as Hanna hobbled back to her seat and looked angrily at the lecturer as if wondering why he had stopped.

That night, at about two in the morning I woke with a start, so full of energy I didn't know what to do with myself. I got up and went downstairs and then outside to sit by the pond and look at the Rocky Mountains silhouetted against the blue-black sky. I suddenly knew that this was the last night that I would ever have Chronic Fatigue and surprisingly, the thought saddened me. I sat quietly, listening to that feeling and I realized how much room CFS had made in my previously too busy life. It had given me almost a year to do nothing but pay attention to myself. Something I never would have done for myself without it. And it had softened my life. It had softened me. And brought me down from too great a height, back to where I touched the earth and the earth touched me. So I sat with the mountains, and the softness and the gentle earth until the tiredness rose up gently, like a small wave on a quiet sea and I went to back to bed, for my last night with CFS.

I awoke the next morning as I had every morning for months, more tired than when I went to sleep. The interlude during the night had gone like a dream or a fairy tale. Mornings were always the worst, because it seemed the one thing that helped with the tiredness was eating, and morning was the longest stretch I went without food. So I took another dose of the B. E. Kit (which by this time I'd learned stood for Epstein Bar - being German, Hanna often puts words in different order than we do in English) and went downstairs to start another day. I had breakfast, morning classes and another dose with lunch and still no change.

After lunch we were in a class about crystals, when it started to happen. I felt it at first like rushes, coffee or fear or joy I couldn't tell which, so I got up and went to experience it alone and with my full and undivided attention. Everything seemed to stand still, as if the world was just a picture and I was an actor on stage with a backdrop of the Rockies and a pond for scenery. And then it happened. I could suddenly feel my reach go out, all the way out into the blackness of space and I could see my energy in little bits of light like stars. A call had gone out and my little energy bits all suddenly woke up all at once and came rushing towards me from every direction and from a great, long distance away, though it only took about two seconds for them all to converge on my body. It made a sound. Like air rushing though a small opening, getting louder and louder, whoosh! And then BANG, my vision cleared up like a lens clicking into focus. And colors, which I hadn't noticed being dulled, became so vivid it was startling! And my body swelled and my blood raced and I could feel the last of the virons racing out towards my skin and leaping out.

It was a miracle and I felt it and saw it and experienced it right as it was happening. It was the miracle that the spirit of the sweat lodge had promised me. It was the miracle that the woman who didn't believe had seen behind me. It was the miracle that I had committed to with the one way ticket. I was cured!

I'd like to say that that was the end of the story, because it'd be nice and neat and friendly that way, but Hanna had told me that a lot of people with chronic fatigue need to take her X-40 kit after starting the B.E. Kit because the virus, according to her, sometimes changes in reaction to the B.E. Kit into something else and the X-40 kit blocks that from happening.

How does the homeopathy work? What I believe is that it is basically the essence - the vibration - of the natural substances from which it is made. And as pure vibration it gently sets up that vibration inside your body. With each dose your system's basic frequency changes by tiny increments to the sum of your body's current frequency, plus this new frequency. And that tiny shift, while imperceptible to our senses, changes the host environment just enough to change your body from a perfect place to settle down and raise a family of CFS virons, to a hell-hole so unpleasant they leave in droves. And that's just what they did.

But with access to the reproductive process, viruses have the ability to mutate and change during reproduction, as AIDS and other viruses have been known to do, and so some of the virons may decide to try an adaptive behavior, instead of exodus. And that's why in my case Hanna suggested that I use the X-40 kit after the B.E. Kit had done its work.

Now I had heard that one of the experiences people sometimes have with homeopathy is that they relive the progression of the disease, backwards during the cure. That didn't happen with the B.E. Kit, but it did with the X-40. I started it about four days after I started the B.E. Kit, about two days after my energy returned. By the second day I began to feel as though I were being dragged back into the illness. At first I went right back to the experience I'd had during my twenty-one days in Colorado. No Commandant but no energy either. It was terrifying, as I'm sure other people with CFS can imagine, because good days and relapses are a part of the roller coaster we are on throughout the disease's course. Some voice inside me kept saying, "See, it was just a fluke, a few good days, but now we're back where we belong." But I knew that wasn't so. I had experienced the miracle and so I just held my fear like the scared little boy it was and sang him to sleep.

As the two weeks worth of B.E. Kit came to an end, I still had about four days worth of X-40 to go. Fortunately I had kept a journal throughout this experience and so I was able to follow the course of the X-40 healing, by literally flipping the pages backwards and seeing where I would be next. As the disease rewound back to the beginning of my illness, I realized that I was going to have to go back into the concentration camp. That was the last lesson. I had one day's worth of X-40 left and that was the only experience I hadn't relived. I had to confront the Commandant one last time.

About the time I had the onset flu, "Schindler's List" was playing in the theaters. I had sworn I would never go see it, because I had lived through it through the disease. But this was different. This was required by my commitment to heal. So the next day, after taking the last dose of X-40, I went to the movies. My grandfather was there. Sitting beside me in the dark, even though he had died more than twenty years before. He had lived through that stunning time of horror, like I had just lived through a tiny fragment of it. And suddenly I understood at a level below words why a "Commandant", and why all the concentration camp images. As an American Jew raised in a pristine suburb, all of that had seemed very far away. Impersonal and general - like history - or a story. That is the white-washing aspect of the American Melting Pot culture. We are untouched by our own history and as a result are unfeeling about our own plight. But CFS had knocked over the pedestal I had lived on, dropped me into the primal ooze of the jungle of my own story and made me live it, live the horror and live the lessons. With CFS, your faith can't be something that you take out every Sunday and dust off like your "go to meeting clothes." It's like survival rations and the ground you walk on. It has muscle and bone, it cuts barbed wire fences like metal shears and it has the force of courage and the will of the righteous.

Grandpa walked along with me as I walked the five miles home from the cinema. He talked to me about his shame for having survived the pogroms and I realized that as a Jew I had inherited his survivor's guilt. And somehow under that blue, blue sky, big enough to cover

149

the Rocky Mountains and still leave room for healing and growing, Grandpa Morris and I got over our guilt. He realized that his surviving was, in part at least, about my life and I realized that my life was in part for him.

And as I climbed the steps of my apartment, I realized that I had just walked five miles and I wasn't even winded.   I fact, I felt like dancing!

Recommended website
www.peacefulmeadowretreat.com

Max Rivers

Susie's Story

Reclaiming me – the *real* me

I had ME for over ten years but it was only diagnosed 2001, after which I tried absolutely everything I could to help myself get better. Although I frequently gained relief from the symptoms for a short while, nothing, absolutely nothing, worked in the long term. This was all the more frustrating for me as a trained Louise Hay 'You Can Heal Your Life', group leader. With my background in understanding, as I thought, metaphysical healing, and my skills as a 'Living Magically' workshop facilitator, I'd healed myself before, so why wasn't I able to this time around? When nothing I tried worked I began to feel powerless and despondent. It was as if the world I knew was crumbling around me and the ground I'd been standing on for so long was now unsafe.

So I just did my best. I meditated. That helped. I went for massages. They helped. I had saunas, which helped to clear out the toxins accumulating in my system, although why I kept feeling so 'poisoned' I couldn't understand. I tried homeopathy, creative visualisation, magnets, kinesiology, reiki, crystal healing, reflexology, emotional freedom techniques, flower remedies, herbalism, energy healing, counselling, cognitive behavioural therapy and even some acupuncture. I ate healthily. I took various supplements and vitamin pills, trying one kind after another. I used pacing, as recommended by our local Chronic Fatigue clinic. I avoided all chemicals. I went swimming and to yoga classes, when I could manage them. I was positive and cheerful. I watched endless funny videos, trying to emulate the work begun by Norman Cousins and which I'd studied further with Robert Holden of the Happiness Project, in Oxford. Most of these things helped, but they only helped to ease the awful symptoms and lessen their impact on my body. They didn't help me get better. I still had ME.

Gradually, over time, my ability to walk diminished and my energy levels dropped to almost zero. Just to get myself showered and dressed took so much energy that I would have to rest watching daytime television, or go back to bed. I had to dish out my energy as if it was a rare and precious commodity. I'd sleep for days to top it up before an appointment. Then afterwards I'd be ill again, often for days. I was in incredible pain and constantly using hot water bottles or co-codemol, or both, to ease that pain. Sometimes it was so bad, I'd be vomiting.

But in between these bouts of dire illness, I didn't look ill! People only believed I was really ill if they saw me at my very worst. That was incredibly frustrating and saddening as I was completely reliant on friends and family for help, just to get by each day.

I read every book I could lay my hands on that offered some small hope of understanding what was going on in my body. My bookshelves were groaning with all those books! I looked into thyroid problems and candida albicans and I investigated the possibility of infectious diseases such as rickettsia. I tried all kinds of special diets that promised to give me more energy, or alleviate or clear the symptoms of whatever it was that I thought it might be. I watched all of the 'You Are What You Eat' programmes on television, and of course, sprouted my own seeds and ate them with my food. I took masses of supplements and vitamin pills. My doctor was very supportive in all of this, but none of the tests showed anything, despite the fact that I had so many symptoms that they filled four sheets of A4 paper!

I had to get food intolerance tests done privately because they weren't available on the NHS, and these tests showed that I was intolerant to some foods. Consequently I was able to remove the offending foods and my digestive problems eased.

Despite all my best efforts on my own behalf I continued to deteriorate. I usually had my food delivered to my door, but if ever I ran out of something and needed to go in person I had to use a walking stick or an electric scooter at Tesco. I even thought about getting a wheelchair or a scooter for myself as my walking was so limited, but I lived on a steep hill with steps up to my front door, so it would have been impractical. I had people coming in to clean, shop and cook for me at least three times a week. I was in a huge amount of debt because, like most others with ME, getting any benefits is a total nightmare and far too costly on our exhausted energy supplies to take to appeal - as we are so often forced to do.

I still had no idea what was causing all my symptoms, which made it all the harder to deal with. I never knew if what I was trying to do to help was in fact making things worse. In March 2005 was my sixtieth birthday and it highlighted just how ill I was. I couldn't celebrate properly, despite wanting to have a big party. I had to see friends and family in small numbers and rest up for days in between. I was completely devastated and wondered if this was how the rest of my life would remain, the prospect was daunting and depressing. I actually began to feel scared for the first time since I realised I had ME.

One day, a friend who had similar symptoms to mine and who was also looking for answers, told me about a special treatment for ME which was being offered locally. At first I scoffed. But then, as Deepak Chopra says, 'coincidences' are never 'accidental' and another friend with similar symptoms also called me. She asked if I'd heard about a treatment for ME called Mickel Therapy, which was being given near where I live. I decided I needed to find out more and after that I made an appointment for some treatment.

At my first session, it was explained to me that according to Dr David Mickel, a former General Practitioner, what we call ME is actually 'hypothalamitis', a dysfunctional hypothalamus, which then creates all the multitude of symptoms so well known to anyone with ME. It explained every single symptom that I had and for the first time I felt totally understood, and hopeful! I started to understand what had been going on in my body at long last. That was such a huge relief. Now I knew what I was up against! We talked about how hypothamalitis first begins; that is, what might have caused my hypothalamus to become dysfunctional. The concept of a 'body-mind', a consciousness that is aware and totally separate from my 'head-mind', was introduced. I'd already read Dr Candace Pert's 'Molecules of Emotion', in which she describes how her scientific trials to find a cure for cancer led to a mind-blowing discovery that each of our cells has its own consciousness and can think for themselves, so the idea of a separate body-mind resonated deeply with me and it all began to make sense. The fact was that this body-mind was 'The Boss' and *not* the head-mind as we are all led to believe.

After my first session I felt 'blasted', but very, very calm, and certain that this form of treatment would help me. What I liked best was that the healing process was completely in my hands. Instead of feeling powerless as I'd done on my sixtieth birthday, I began to feel quietly confident in my own body's ability to heal, if I listened to and acted upon the subtle messages it was giving me. All I needed to do was translate those messages into appropriate, constructive, healthy, actions on my own behalf. My therapist's job in all of this was to help me find the message my body had been trying to send me and to then keep me on track so that I remained true to my body's needs, rather than those of my head-mind. And that, I discovered as I made my own healing journey, was the hardest part!

Mickel Therapy blew me away simply because it was so very different to anything else. I was completely taken with the concept that our body-mind sends us information in the form of e-motions and that if we listen to them and take appropriate action they dissipate and disappear. If we ignore them however, as we often do in our Western culture, then the message from our body-mind becomes much louder and develops into symptoms. By then our body-mind really has our attention!

Unfortunately, we are so unused to hearing and translating these messages that we don't realise they are helpful. Instead we try to avoid them or remove them in some way, often with medication or other prescribed courses of action like 'pacing', or CBT, or even relaxation. What I did, when feeling so very ill and utterly exhausted beyond endurance, was, not unnaturally, take some pills for the pain and then sleep until I felt better.

I loved the idea that Mickel Therapy placed my healing in my own hands, as I'm a firm believer in the power of the individual. I'd also suspected for a long time that my illness had something to teach me, but until finding Mickel Therapy I had no idea what that lesson was. I began to realise that I could trust my body-mind and all the feelings it sent me in much the same way that I would often trust my instincts about situations - and they would usually turn out to be spot on.

The more I trusted in my body-mind the more I got better. I decided to take more care of myself. I got my hair done and bought new clothes so that I wasn't still living in my comfortable old sweat shirt and jogging trousers. My energy returned and I felt fantastic. My therapist made me challenge others in my life and stand up for myself. This was incredibly scary and stressful for me, but I did it as best as I could. When I didn't manage to do it she told me that was why I was still ill. Naturally, I thought my therapist was wonderful, so I kept on trying! She even suggested that I do the training. So I applied for it, and was accepted.

However, as time went by and I began to find my own feet, I had to challenge my therapist and this did not turn out to be a positive experience. In fact, I had already started to become more and more ill again and her inability to explain why, or help, had left me alone in continuing Mickel Therapy. None of the many messages she had given me, the messages she translated as coming from my body-mind, worked. I began to realise none of them ever had. What I'd done was do my best to listen and act for myself. The more my therapist urged me to do what she thought I should do, the more ill I became, and the less she was able to help, until she became a part of the problem.

Eventually I became so ill and so desperate that I appealed to Dr Mickel himself, as I truly believed in his ideas, and he worked with me. With his guidance I soon got back on track again and rapidly regained my health. His approach was completely different from my former therapist, he encouraged me to trust in myself, not him! As they had never helped me we scrapped all the messages that my former therapist had given me and worked instead with Dr Mickel's newest development, the 'Keys for Health'. He also taught me how to do my 'Notes',a four step process of working with the Keys for Health that helped me to understand for myself whether or not the actions I was taking were actually helping, or weren't. With David guiding me, I soon regained my own inner trust in myself and my body-mind. I re-learned how to work out for myself what my body-mind was trying to communicate and how to live my life in co-operation, not competition with it, a process I was familiar with from my Living Magically work. It was often very challenging and very hard work, but it was all worth it, because it's given me back myself, and I've learned what I need to do to remain true to myself.

Now I'm feeling really great, thanks to Dr. David Mickel. I think the best part is that I no longer have any food intolerances and of course, I can drink the odd glass of red wine (or G and T!) with no nasty after effects at all – yippee! More than just feeling better, I feel *empowered*. I now have the tools to keep me well. If I do become unwell again, I can simply use them, learn from the experience, and develop my skills of listening to the whispers of my body-mind even better. This has given me incredible confidence and a much more balanced and joyful life. Oh, and of course I completed my training and I'm now a fully qualified Mickel Therapist. I did some further studying and am now also a fully qualified Life and Performance Coach, helping people achieve success in their lives, which fits in well with my Mickel Therapy. And I am loving it all!

I've regained my health, and so much more. I'm starting to catch up on the huge, huge, mountain of stuff that got pushed to one side for later, each time I became too ill to cope. Slowly, I'm getting my finances, and the home I was too ill to do anything to, in order. Slowly, I'm getting there! Now I can begin to catch up on my life, and all the things I've had to sideline for years and years. I've learned to be more emotionally honest,with myself, and with others. I've learned to meet my own needs first and not last, although catching myself falling into the trap of putting others first is often the hardest part! I'm starting to discover, at the ripe old age of sixty-one, just what it is that I really want to do with my life. I look at photos of myself when I was ill and can see how drained, ill and old I looked and how there was no-one at home behind my eyes. I was in too much pain. At long last I'm at home in my own body, my spirit is returning and I'm learning how to be a part of the human race again. But I'm taking life at my own pace, not at the pace my head-mind tells me I ought to take.

Thank you so much David Mickel. I know you told me, when I last thanked you, that you didn't need my thanks as I'd done all the work myself. It's true I did, and it was damned hard work and often very uncomfortable. Frequently it required a great deal of courage as I made changes in my life, I'll admit that. It still isn't easy as I continue to apply the 'keys to my health' to my life on a daily basis. But you haven't just given me back my life Dr Mickel, you've given me back more of who I really am, the real ME. That is the greatest gift of all.

It's time the NHS started to take notice of just how effective this treatment is. And how cost effective too. Without resorting to drugs or special diets I've regained my health and my freedom.

Well done Dr David Mickel!

Most useful aid to recovery - Mickel Therapy

Recommended book - "The Long Awaited Cure" by Dr David Mickel.

Recommended website - www.mickeltherapy.com

Susie Novis

Alex's Story

My journey from ME to health and happiness

Up until the age of sixteen I was in many ways like most teenagers. I lived for three things: music, sport, and the opposite sex. School and homework were just something that had to be done to free up my time to embark upon these three passions. Like everyone I had heard about illnesses such as ME and CFS, but the idea of something like that happening to me was not something I would have dreamed of. Spending seven years suffering from a severely debilitating chronic illness was about as likely as being on the next space shuttle to the moon and back.

Towards the end of my GCSEs I started to become tired and ended up in bed for several weeks with a bad virus, but this was hardly surprising. As far as I, the doctor, and my family were concerned, I just needed to rest for a while and I would be able to get back to enjoying the summer as usual. Ignorance really is bliss.

Three months later only really one thing had changed, I had another three months of practice for an uncertain, and at times almost unbearable, future under my belt. Tired of being unable to do anything, I made a desperate attempt to start at Sixth Form. Willpower got me through about ten days, before almost collapsing and spending weeks in bed just getting to the point that I could leave the house for a few minutes again. Struggling to get from the bedroom to the bathroom and back, and fit in a small amount of schoolwork became my daily struggle for the next two years. I quickly lost contact with my girlfriend, my friends, my hobbies, and in many ways the person I took to be myself.

After two years of living hell I reached the point that I simply couldn't take anymore. I'd already made major changes in my nutrition, which had included eating no sugar, yeast, wheat, preservatives or flavourings for the past two years. I had been to see numerous health practitioners, both conventional and otherwise, and still nothing had really changed. Depression was certainly not the cause of my miserable existence, but it was undoubtedly an inevitable consequence. As far as I was concerned it was looking like my life was over.

Just as I reached rock bottom, I called my Uncle to tell him how I felt. In essence, I hated my life and everything about it. His response was very different to the typical response you might get in this situation. Rather than giving me sympathy or telling me that it would all be alright, he offered me something far more important. He asked me a series of life changing questions. The first of which was, "On a scale of 0-10, how badly do you want things to change?" After thinking about this for a few minutes, and deciding that I wouldn't shoot somebody, and I wouldn't chop off my arm, I came to the conclusion that I was probably a nine and a half out of ten, I would do virtually anything to change my situation. My Uncle then asked me to make a list of all the things I thought I could do to change my situation, to which I added things like learning more about nutrition, practicing meditation and yoga on a consistent basis, learning how to get my mind into the right state to support my healing, and learning more about complementary health. My Uncle then asked me to list all the things that I felt made me worse. I had only one thing on this list: life. Just getting through the day felt like a major struggle on a daily basis.

After spending some time discussing these ideas, my Uncle asked me a question that really made me think. The question was, "How many hours a day do you spend doing the things you yourself believe could make a difference?" The answer to this question was virtually none. So here I was, I wanted my life to change more than virtually anything, I had a rough idea of things I could do to change my situation, but I was consistently doing virtually nothing about it. My Uncle then asked me how many hours a day I spent watching television. The answer was about seven. Television had become my friend, it was the one thing that I could do that didn't require any real physical energy, and it meant that I could go off into another world and ignore the reality of my life. At the age of eighteen years old I virtually had a PhD in soap operas. This was hardly the vision I had had for my life.

Over the next hour or so, my Uncle helped me come up with a daily plan of how I could start to integrate my list of potentially helpful strategies into my daily routine. The commitments that I made included never watching more than two hours of television a day, doing thirty minutes meditation a day, five minutes yoga, starting to consistently read books on health and psychology, finding a meditation teacher, and to find a therapist to help look at my psychology. For me at this point, I was too ill to sit in a chair and meditate for thirty minutes, so I would lie in a garden recliner kept in my bedroom to do so. My five minutes of yoga was really just doing yoga breathing, as I felt too weak to do any postures. However, I did have one essential resource; I was so desperate that I approached my commitments like my life depended upon them. I guess in many ways it did.

I soon realised that one of the things I needed were positive role models. Essentially, people who had been through similar experiences to mine and found a way out, as the negativity around ME was becoming all consuming. Struggling to find stories of people who had recovered from ME I went in search of people who had recovered from other serious conditions.

One story I came across had a particularly powerful impact upon me, this was the story of Meir Schneider. Meir was born blind, and after a number of failed operations in his early years, he was told there was no way he would ever be able to see. In his teenage years, Meir decided there was a whole world that he was missing out on, and that he would therefore do everything he could to find a way to see. Of course people around him thought he was either in denial or delusional, but Meir had a strength of spirit far beyond your average teenager. One of the techniques that Meir came across was a technique called palming, which effectively involves staring at the sun with closed eyes, and slowly covering and uncovering your closed eyes with your hands. How many minutes in the average day do you think you could do this for before you became really, really, bored? Five minutes? Fifteen minutes? Meir used to do this technique for five hours a day, every single day. His level of commitment and resilience was in a league of its own. Several years later, through this, and a number of other techniques, Meir's eyesight was virtually normal. Meir's story taught me something fundamental: if I was willing to give everything I could to my recovery, even though I could not yet see how it was possible, with persistence and perseverance perhaps I would find a way.

After six months of my new plan, and only marginal improvements, a new challenge unfolded for me: school. I was three months away from my A-levels, and having spent three years studying for them, I was still massively behind. The problem was that I needed A-levels to get to university, which to me seemed like the perfect answer. I mean what do students do all day? They sleep! Finally I was going to find somewhere that I would fit in! Secondly, students get student loans, and that was going to mean £15,000 to spend on my health.

At the school I attempted to attend, there was this joke about 'The Myth of Alex Howard,' because I was hardly ever seen there. On one of the few afternoons I had been able to make it to class, the deputy headmaster spotted me walking through the school yard, and took what was a rare opportunity to have a word with me. He told me that considering how far behind I was, he felt it probably wasn't worth me continuing. As part of what I had been reading to attempt to turn my health around, I had been reading a lot about the power of the mind to focus on something and make the impossible happen. Considering it was taking some time to turn my health around, I figured that perhaps this might be a good opportunity to test out this idea. The goal I set was to get straight A's in my A-levels, something that virtually no one achieves, especially considering my subjects were History, Economics and Business Studies, by no means easy subjects.

I spent the three months prior to my exams doing everything I could to teach myself all that I had missed. I only had about three hours a day that I was able to work for, so in these three hours I had to be totally focused, and I found that a number of accelerated learning techniques also made a big difference. Over these three months I taught myself a huge amount of work, and I caught up considerably. Unfortunately I pushed myself too hard. A week before my exams I had a major relapse.

I did end up taking my exams, but it took me four hours to do each three-hour exam. I would write my first essay over the allowed forty-five minutes. I would then lay in the bed next to my desk (I was taking my exams in the school's sick room) for twenty minutes until I was awoken by my supervisor. Then I would write an essay for another forty-five minutes. I would then sleep for twenty minutes. I would then write for forty-five minutes, sleep for another twenty minutes, and finally finish the exam. This was a rather painstaking way of doing it, but even this was an incredible strain on me, and to this day I have very little recollection of this whole period.

When I got my A-level results I got a very rude awakening. A rude awakening to the true power of the human spirit. I had achieved my goal. I got straight As, along with the highest marks in the school in some of my papers. This greatly strengthened my resolve, and I got back to working intensely on turning around my health for another three years.

These three years at university were the period where I really went on my journey with true conviction. Every minute I was awake was about understanding my health and self. I read over five hundred books on all different kinds of psychology, spirituality, energy work, hypnosis, meditation, health, and anything else that might hold the answers to my inner journey. Much of the time was incredibly lonely, for there was often no one that I could share my experiences or journey with.

Yet, something else that I learned is that it is in the deepest loneliness and pain that we hear the most important voice of all: the voice of our soul and spirit, and it was this that I constantly aligned myself with.

There were times when I read a passage in a book that would touch me on a profound level, and because I had no one to share it with, in some ways it touched me even more deeply. I spent countless hours in meditation and practicing yoga, and as my health slowly returned I started to go for longer and longer walks along Swansea Bay, dragging my frail body with unstoppable determination a few steps further each time.

At the end of these three years I earned a first class degree in psychology (for which I had won the Best Student Award from the British Psychological Society), as well as getting an advanced diploma in clinical hypnotherapy, neuro-linguistic programming and life coaching (I did my post-graduate training at the same time as the third year of my degree – quadrupling my reading speed had made studying a lot easier). Far more important than this was the fact that I had been able to take great strides forward in my health. Upon leaving university I went into practice with my teacher in hypnotherapy and moved to London. It seemed that the more I learned about human psychology, the more changes I was able to make in my life.

Another six months later, and I had made a full recovery. Like most people who are seriously ill, I had a benchmark that once I reached I knew I had made it. For me this was to be able to go for a run with no ill effects afterwards. This was something I had dreamed about doing for seven years, and to say it was an amazing feeling is perhaps the greatest understatement possible.

In the four years since then, a whole new journey has opened up and unfolded. With the publication of my auto-biographical story, 'WHY ME? My Journey from M.E. to Health and Happiness,' and the results I was starting to get in The Optimum Health Clinic working with other sufferers, I soon found myself inundated with people seeking help on their own healing journeys. I quickly brought on board a clinical nutritionist, and the clinic since then has grown from strength to strength. It has now worked with over one thousand people with ME and even has clinical trials being launched by a top London university.

Being fully recovered is a strange experience. In a DVD we recently made about patient experiences at the clinic, one of the interviewees described it as being on one hand totally amazing, and on the other hand totally natural. I think that is a really good description. There are times when I'm reminded how much energy I now have (like when I've had work experience people with me begging to have a lie in because they are struggling to keep up with my schedule!) and yet living life at one-hundred miles an hour just seems so natural and an expression of who I am.

Most useful aid to recovery - having an integrative approach such as The Optimum Health Clinic now uses (see 'More About The Authors' at the back of the book).

Alex Howard

Karen's Story

The Mossop Philosophy changed my life

Looking back now I am certain it all started when I was at school. I recollect a teacher accusing me of skiving and I remember feeling quite upset that she didn't believe I was genuinely ill with another bad throat. This was over twenty-five years ago, but I was actually diagnosed with CFS approximately thirteen years later. At the time of diagnosis I think I got it quite mildly. I was constantly suffering with throat infections, tonsillitis, vertigo and viruses, which made me ache all over so much that it hurt to move. My throat would swell up so badly that I could hardly talk or eat. There were even times when I thought my airways would completely block due to the swelling. Sometimes these illnesses made me so ill that I was admitted to hospital. Eventually I was referred to the Infectious Diseases Clinic where I was diagnosed with CFS.

I had lost one job due to my bad health, but at the time of diagnosis I was working full-time for the Local Authority. They were very good about me frequently having to take time off sick but I used to feel bad about constantly letting my team down, so in 1996 I decided to take a step down and moved within the Local Authority to a less stressful job.

At the same time as the job change I decided to slow down the pace of my life. I changed my lifestyle. I learned how to meditate and I kept stress levels to a minimum. My health gradually started to improve and eventually I believed the ME had gone for good. I thought it had left me weaker than other people, as I still caught every virus going around and I still took longer to get better than others, but apart from that I was managing to live a normal life.

In 1998 I got married and in 2000 I became a mum. My health continued to improve and was fairly good until the end of 2002 when I was pregnant with my second child.

The hospital where I was due to give birth caused me a great deal of stress and I caught a 'flu' type virus in December which lasted until March 2003, after the delivery of my second son. In May that year we put our house up for sale and I endured another period of prolonged stress. We moved into rented accommodation in September and then eventually into our new home in October. Just weeks later in November 2003 I thought I had flu. With two small children to look after I couldn't rest and instead dosed myself up with paracetamol, ibuprofen and aspirin, and struggled on. This 'flu' dragged on for months. A friend suggested that perhaps the ME had returned but I dismissed the idea. At that time I knew very little about ME and I really thought that I no longer had it, believing that it was impossible to 'catch' ME again!

By March 2004 I was confined to bed. I could barely walk. I could just about manage to go to the bathroom and back, approximately twenty steps in total, and I hurt all over. Every muscle and every joint was painful, and although I tried all sorts of over the counter pain relief, none of them seemed to help at all. I lay in bed for two weeks and despite being so dreadfully tired I couldn't sleep. All I could do was lie there and look at either the ceiling or the wall hoping that I'd eventually fall asleep and wake up feeling a little better. But of course this didn't happen. It was horrendous and I felt so isolated. I was incredibly weak and so desperately ill that I thought I was going to die. My children had to go to full-time nursery or to relatives to be looked after.

I was taken to see my doctor (GP) who suggested blood tests to investigate further. They all came back negative. One test came back showing that I'd had glandular fever in the past, just as it did years ago when I was diagnosed with ME by the Infectious Diseases Clinic. My GP confirmed the illness was ME. I was devastated, it felt as if my whole world had been torn apart – how on earth could I be a mother when I couldn't even look after myself?

I was extremely fortunate to have a very supportive husband and family who were caring for me. My parents would come over to give my husband some respite. They also tried hard to find out what alternative medicines could help me. They suggested healing and herbs. I saw a local healer which did help slightly, as afterwards I was no longer confined to bed and could manage the stairs, but I still couldn't do much. I tried to spoon-feed my one-year-old son but found that even this small task was too strenuous for me, and I ended up lying back on the sofa again.

At the end of March I went to see a herbalist at a well-known herbal clinic in Leicester. I was convinced that this would be my cure. I did everything that she recommended. I had complete bed rest and took the tinctures three times a day.

I started to improve and by June I returned to my part-time job on a very part-time basis. I would have stopped working altogether, but I was allowed to return on therapeutic hours working up to six hours a week, instead of the usual sixteen.

I learned how to pace and the herbal medication boosted my immune system and kept any depression away. I was now functioning at about 50%. I was able to walk for approximately twenty minutes without a break, do a bit of shopping, cook a meal and drive the car, but I couldn't do anything too exhausting like vacuuming, ironing or running around with the children.

At the beginning of October I had a set back. I wasn't as ill as I was in the March but even so I was unable to do much. I remember even struggling to take off my coat. I was feeling dreadful, my throat was swollen and I was exhausted and aching all over again. It wasn't until the end of October that I was functioning back at about 50%.

My dad heard about a healer in London named Sonia who had achieved some astonishing results, so when I was feeling a bit better he took me to see her. Luckily he has a very comfortable car so I was able to rest on the way. Sonia's healing was powerful and I did feel the benefits for a few days afterwards. She told me about an amazing lady called Professor Diana Mossop who, she felt certain, would be able to help me. Sonia explained that all I was doing was masking the symptoms with the herbal medication and that what was needed was to pinpoint the virus and obliterate it, which she was certain Professor Mossop would be able to do. Sonia explained that Professor Mossop uses phytobiophysics to treat patients, and although she herself had some basic training in phytobiophysics, she felt sure my needs would be best met if I saw Professor Mossop herself.

I took her advice and booked an appointment in London with Professor Mossop.

At the end of June my dad again chauffeured me down to London. We were very excited about the appointment and as we pulled up outside the clinic I was quite nervous and I remember thinking that this could be it, my life could be totally changed and I was so hoping that it would.

The appointment lasted for just one hour. Professor Mossop was so lovely and welcoming and I was soon at ease. She explained that ME wasn't a disease, it was a blanket term for symptoms where the cause is unknown. I then put my left foot on a small metal plate and my other foot on her lap. Professor Mossop used a small machine which measures frequency. A probe was attached to this machine with which she touched my big toe on my right foot. She explained that the body vibrates at a certain frequency, as do viruses. I was informed that my energy levels were very low and she then asked me to lay my hand across several bottles at a time. If the needle on the machine went too high or too low then I had to touch each individual bottle to see which one was causing the problem. There were a lot of these bottles to touch and the whole hour was predominantly spent going through all of these.

At the end of all these tests Professor Mossop found glandular fever, polio, meningitis and mercury poisoning in my system. She also found a minor heart problem which I'd forgotten about, which amazed me as I'd had tests done at the Leicester Royal Infirmary years ago and nothing was found. The meningitis and polio were due to vaccinations and the mercury poisoning was due to a leaky filling.

I was advised to have the filling replaced with a white filling and in time replace the other four amalgam fillings, with four monthly intervals between each one as it would be far too dangerous to replace them all together. I was given four bottles of medicine and a Heartlock and Journey Analysis form which showed dates of traumas throughout my life for me to look at. Out of the four bottles of medicine one contained a liquid and the other three bottles contained pills for the viruses.

I purchased a Phytobiophysics Superfit Formula and Phytobiophysics Flower Formula and also the following supplements: Pharma Nord Super Bio-Quinone Q10, Pharma Nord Bio-Pycnogenol, Herbs of Grace Aller-G and Lifestream Bioactive Spirulina.

I was advised to stay clear of citrus, white wine, pork and crab meat and to come back in six weeks. It was all very relaxed, matter of fact and very simple.

I came out feeling extremely tired. I had been struggling to concentrate and take in all of the information she was telling me. I feel awful saying this now but at the time I felt a bit suspicious and disappointed. The appointment wasn't what I expected. It all seemed much too simple. I'd been suffering for years with ME and here was Professor Mossop saying that it was all these other viruses causing the illness. How on earth could she diagnose this in just one hour when our so called 'health professionals' couldn't in all these years? I felt very sceptical and was actually feeling quite despondent about the whole appointment. I had looked at the Heartlock and Journey Analysis form showing the dates of traumas I had experienced and at that time couldn't make any sense of it. I was exhausted and when I got back into my dad's car I tried my hardest to sound enthusiastic about the whole thing. He had taken time out of work, driven me all the way down to London and paid for the appointment and I didn't want him to feel let down as he too was sure that Professor Mossop would cure me. It was very difficult trying to sound positive when I really felt inside that it had been a waste of time and money.

I waited until Friday when the supplements arrived from Jersey before I started taking the new medication and stopped taking the herbal medicine I was using. Late afternoon I cooked a meal using a jar of sauce which I normally use, had a normal relaxing evening and went to bed. That night I woke up at about 3am with awful stomach pains. It was my irritable bowel syndrome starting up again, so I came downstairs and took some Colofac pills and Gaviscon. I went back to bed but was unable to sleep due to the pain. At 4am I came downstairs again and sat on the sofa. I eventually fell asleep and at 6am when my husband came downstairs with the children I returned to bed for a couple of hours. When I woke up I wondered if the sauce I used for the meal contained any of the things I had been advised to avoid. When I looked at the label on the sauce I discovered there was lemon juice in the ingredients. Obviously in the past the herbal medication had prevented such reactions as I used this same sauce on a regular basis without any problems. When I got up at 8am I was surprised at how awake I felt. Normally after a bad night I would have a set back, however I seemed to be OK. I wondered if it was due to the new medication I was taking, but dismissed this idea as I was quite sure it wasn't going to work.

On the following Sunday I still felt okay, in fact slightly better than usual and when I went to bed that night it was much later than usual.

On the Monday I woke up feeling fantastic. I felt really energised and I could think clearly. My usual aches and pains had disappeared and I even looked different. I went to work for the usual few hours and was told I looked 'radiant' and 'really well'. I didn't know what to say to these comments. I couldn't say I felt fantastic in case it didn't last! It was amazing and I realised that it was more than a coincidence. The Mossop Philosophy was working. I couldn't remember ever feeling so well. It was a miracle! That evening my husband and I celebrated with a bottle of rosé wine and raised our glasses to Professor Mossop.

The following morning I woke feeling awful again, I couldn't believe it. I remember thinking that I was right after all, the medicine wouldn't work. It was dreadful having experienced 'life' the day before to again feeling so unwell. About half way though that day I remembered Professor Mossop had advised to stay away from white wine, which I had forgotten about. I was told so much in that one hours' appointment and as I was feeling so drained at the time it was difficult to remember everything I had been told. Of course, the rosé wine contained white wine. It took a few days to get back to feeling great again and by the Friday of that same week I was again feeling fantastic.

From then I just kept on getting better and better and I was thinking about ending my pacing routine. I had cut my rest periods from two hours down to half an hour per day. I felt I couldn't stop my rests completely as I was afraid of a relapse, but on the fourth week of feeling good I took my sons out for the day and was unable to rest.

The following day I had a dental and hospital appointment and I didn't manage to rest that day either and on the day after that we were going on holiday and I had to finish the packing which took most of the day, so I again didn't get a chance to rest.

I had now missed three days in a row of resting and I still felt good. I knew by now that this feeling great was here to stay and just in time for my holiday! We all had a great holiday and when we got back I returned to see Professor Mossop for my follow-up appointment.

My energy levels were again measured and although they weren't as good as they should have been they were double those of the previous visit. I told her how good I felt and she did some more tests. The tests showed that I no longer had any of the polio, meningitis or glandular fever viruses or mercury poisoning. Some rubella was found and I was given some more pills. I was also advised that I no longer needed the previous tablets prescribed and only to finish some of the supplements. I asked if I should renew any of the new medication once it was finished but was told that it wouldn't be necessary. Professor Mossop said that I wouldn't need to see her again regarding the ME as it wouldn't return. She advised that I could phone her in October/November for some formulas for my family and me to keep flu viruses away and was advised to read as much as possible about nutrition and to get plenty of exercise and to enjoy my new life! I came out of the clinic this time on cloud nine.

It was a true miracle - the ME had finally gone forever!

Since then my life has got better and better. It is now over two years since my recovery. I am still feeling great, very much alive and loving life. I appreciate my good health in a way that I believe you can only do so once you've experienced being so ill for so long. I now walk on average two miles a day which I really enjoy, even if it is raining! And although I thought I ate well before, I now eat a really good, balanced, organic diet.

I am working sixteen hours a week as well as looking after my children and maintaining the household chores, and I am also attending college for two evenings a week. We have additionally undergone quite a stressful house renovation over the past twenty-two months, which I have project managed.

My family and my life are now totally enriched. It is so great having my independence back and not having to rely on my husband and parents to help me with the children and household chores. I am now able to be the mother I always dreamed of being, as I can run around with my children and have a lot of fun with them. Words cannot describe how good that feels. It's truly amazing how the Mossop Philosophy has changed my life! Obviously we are eternally grateful for the Mossop Philosophy and there isn't a day that goes by that I don't fully appreciate and enjoy. Sometimes the sense of being alive and well is overwhelming and I feel so fortunate, overjoyed and at times elated to be living life

A strange thing happened a couple of weeks ago – both my husband and I caught a cold. Normally my husband would recover very quickly and I would stay ill for weeks and be much worse than him even though

we had the same virus. This time it was different. I felt unwell for just a few days and my husband is still feeling ill over two weeks later…..
miracles can definitely happen!

Most useful aid to recovery - the Mossop Philosophy, good nutrition and rest

Recommended websites - www.phytob.com

Karen's advice - don't ever think you won't recover from ME because it is definitely possible.

Karen Hallam

Chris's Story

I knew diet was crucial to my health

My own battle with chronic fatigue syndrome began in 1977 when most doctors had never heard of the condition. Thus I began a lonely, frustrating, and very expensive, journey to alternative practitioners, trying one suggested cure after another and getting no better. In fact, it would be fair to say that almost everything I tried made me worse.

So how did I get well? Well, it was a journey - a journey which is still not fully completed and never will be, because health is something which we only have from day to day. We have to be vigilant about our health, especially when our bodies have been weakened by something like chronic fatigue syndrome. But the good news is this. If you are now sick, you can get well.

Exactly when it started is hard to pinpoint. Perhaps it was as far back as January 1976 when I fainted suddenly one morning while visiting a friend. I had slept badly the previous night and had not eaten breakfast, so I attributed the fainting episode to the combined effects of tiredness and hunger. But for several days afterwards I had a bad headache. Feelings of faintness would come over me at unexpected moments and I feared I might pass out again. Over a period of weeks, the headache lifted and the feelings of faintness became less frequent. But something had changed. I did not feel quite well and seemed increasingly susceptible to colds and sore throats, even in summer.

Until then I had always prided myself on my physical fitness. I was a competitive runner during school and university, training up to sixty miles a week by the time I was eighteen or nineteen, with long runs of more than twenty miles on Sunday mornings. When I graduated from university and started work with the New Zealand public service at the end of 1975, I found less time for serious training although I still ran several times a week and regarded myself as fit.

After the fainting episode my energy for running seemed to wane. I would go out occasionally and run three or four miles, struggling to complete the distance, my legs feeling strangely wooden. "I'm just unfit," I told myself.

At the end of 1976 I moved to Wellington with my job and lived for several weeks in a hostel eating irregular meals. I seemed to have an increased craving for chocolate bars and similar snacks, particularly after work in the early evening as I walked home. I moved into a flat in Hataitai, a hilly Wellington suburb overlooking the sea. Walking uphill from the bus-stop to the flat each evening became increasingly difficult, but I put it down the fact that I was unfit and determined I would get back to regular running again. A series of colds and sore throats put paid to that idea.

In April 1977 my life took a radical new direction. I resigned my job and went to Pakistan to stay with some missionary friends in Hyderabad. I had been interested in overseas missionary work for some time and wondered whether it might be my eventual calling, so the purpose of my trip was to see first-hand the conditions in which missionaries lived and worked.

Before leaving New Zealand I had the usual jabs for cholera, typhoid and malaria. The after-effects of injections left me feeling under par, and when I arrived in Pakistan I felt as though I had a bad cold, which I couldn't throw off.

The heat in Hyderabad was intense. I did a lot of walking around the crowded city and always returned exhausted to my host's house, usually sleeping in the afternoons, as was the local custom. I had a craving for sweets. One way to satisfy it, along with the thirst created by the heat, was to drink several bottles of soft drink each day, usually a local brand called Apple Cidra and sometimes Coca Cola. I also found myself buying packets of Pakistani-style biscuits and eating the whole bag in one sitting.

About two months into my visit, I developed what I thought was the 'flu. I put it down to the heat and the fact that I had been over-exerting myself, and decided to have an early night in the hope of sleeping it off. The next morning when I climbed out of bed, all my strength seemed to have vanished. I felt as weak as a kitten, drained of energy and barely able to walk to the bathroom. I sank back into bed. For several days I spent most of my time asleep and my hosts became increasingly concerned, urging me to see a doctor, which I did. I managed to drag myself to the surgery of a Pakistani doctor who stunned me by suggesting I might have diabetes. Blood tests a few days later showed my blood sugar levels were normal, much to my relief.

Over the next few weeks, my energy slowly returned. I moved to Karachi where I lived in a flat above the home of an English engineer, sharing the flat with two Pakistani students. One morning, I awoke feeling weak and trembling, with a bad headache. I was planning to visit someone in hospital and although I did not feel well, decided to go anyway, in the hope I would 'come right' as the day went on.

I survived the hospital visit - just - and was about to climb onto the back of my friend's motor scooter to return home when I fainted. I came to, lying on the footpath, with a sea of puzzled Pakistani faces looking down at me. It was an awful experience. My friend was panic-stricken when I collapsed. Fearing the worst he ran to his father-in-law's house about a hundred metres away to get help. I managed to walk back to the aforementioned house and collapsed onto a bed for several hours. Thus began three humiliating years of being unable to work at a full-time job. Three years of being misunderstood and being accused of being a malingerer by family and friends who did not understand the constant pain and exhaustion I was battling.

My faith in the medical profession quickly evaporated as several doctors told me there was nothing wrong with me. My blood tests were all 'normal'. Furthermore, I didn't look sick. I was lean and suntanned, and, as one friend put it, I looked "as fit as a buck rabbit". The general consensus among the doctors I visited was that my problems were all in my mind. Somehow, I managed to hang on to my faith in God. I prayed for an answer, and the first glimmer of hope came about three months after I returned to New Zealand when a friend suggested my problems could be caused by food allergies. A few weeks later I was sitting in the consulting room of a food allergy specialist in Wellington. His nurse gave me a series of skin tests to find the foods I was allergic to. She came up with about thirty, including wheat, dairy products, eggs, citrus fruit, potatoes, apples and corn. Essentially, they were all the foods I ate most of.

I had to totally change my diet. Initially, it was a source of much amusement amongst my flatmates, who turned up their noses at the transparent-looking tapioca I was eating for breakfast and the bread made from whiter-than-white gluten-free flour. It all tasted pretty insipid. But I was determined I was going to get well and followed the allergy specialist's instructions to the letter. I was encouraged initially by the disappearance of my acne within a few days on the new diet. That was nothing short of miraculous I thought.

During this time, I was studying Business Administration at Canterbury University but found it increasingly difficult to concentrate on my work. I eventually quit the course at the start of the final term and worked as a part-time gardener for a few months, and then as a part-time window cleaner. The outdoor work was easier on my aching head, but my energy was so low that I could not work a full day. Often, I collapsed into bed exhausted and aching all over.

However, there remained within me a burning desire to get well. The more knock-backs I experienced the more determined I became. The source of my indomitable spirit was largely my faith in God which never wavered, even in the darkest moments, and I clung to Bible verses I had memorised which promised answers to prayer, even if they might be a while coming. I believed without a shadow of doubt that eventually I would get well.

I started reading extensively about nutrition. I devoted my days to studying nutrition and with my limited money I could not afford to buy many books, so I searched libraries for information and browsed in bookshops. Being a fast reader, I could often absorb an entire book within thirty minutes, standing in the shop. I still believed my problem was food allergies. The general consensus among the authors I read was that food allergies were caused by 'stress' and the need for extra vitamins and minerals was also a common theme.

I met my wife, Angie, in October 1981 and we were married in May 1982. Life was wonderful. But I didn't know then that several more years of poor health lay ahead of me. We moved to England where my parents had returned a few years previously, along with my two younger brothers and a sister. I got a job with a London book publisher. Despite suffering bad headaches most afternoons and coming home exhausted at night, I managed to hold down the job, but I knew I could not keep living that way.

Once again, I turned to the study of nutrition in an effort to get well. I read about macrobiotics, food combining, vegetarianism, Ayurvedic medicine, the Pritikin diet and many more theories, experimenting with each in turn. This was much to the frustration of my poor wife whose patience was tested to the limit as she cooked the various meals I requested.

Then I read about hypoglycaemia - low blood sugar. Hypoglycaemia is a major cause of chronic fatigue and some experts believe up to 20% of adults in the western world suffer from the condition. Hypoglycemia is caused by over-activity of the pancreas, which produces too much insulin when sugar or sweet foods are eaten. This over-abundance of insulin metabolises not only the sugar which has been eaten but also some of the glucose which was already present in the bloodstream. The result is a state of low blood sugar which can cause an alarming number of distressing symptoms including fatigue, headaches, dizziness, feeling faint, irritability, depression, difficulty in remembering, blurred vision and in most cases an overwhelming craving for something sweet or a stimulant such as tea or coffee.

The cure, the books said, was to avoid sugar and simple carbohydrates like honey and fruit juice. Caffeine and alcohol were also factors, according to most experts. Now this made sense. I had known instinctively for several years that sweets and coffee made me feel bad, yet in all my nutritional studies I had overlooked the obvious. Perhaps it was because I had always loved sweet things. Not only cakes and biscuits, but healthful natural things like dried fruit, fruit juice and honey.

In my days as a runner I had learned to stoke up on carbohydrates for energy. I had become addicted to sweet things. Now, I started to see light at the end of the tunnel. After a few days of avoiding sweet things, my energy started to come back, my headaches got less and I felt a new sense of vitality. Then I had a particularly stressful day at work and came home exhausted. I craved something sweet. I knew I shouldn't but I couldn't stop myself bingeing on half a dozen muesli bars. Next morning, I woke feeling rotten. It was just like a hangover. I was back to square one again my discouraged mind told me. But I now knew the answer. Be careful with sugar. As long as I kept away from sweets, my energy and health came back, slowly but surely.

Recently a concept known as the 'Glycaemic index' of foods has been developed. The glycaemic index represents the amount by which a food raises the blood sugar level, with glucose having an index of 100. It is interesting that foods such as white bread can raise the blood sugar almost as much as ordinary white sugar, whereas whole-grain breads cause a much slower rise in blood sugar. I proved this myself before I knew anything about glycaemic indexes. When I was experimenting with the high-carbohydrate, low-fat diets I often had a white bread roll with a small amount of low-fat cheese (no butter) and salad for lunch. I would always get a headache during the afternoon following such lunches but I persisted because I thought it was a 'healthy' low-fat meal and it had no sugar. Occasionally, I would have a thick cheese sandwich on wholemeal bread, with butter, and a glass of milk - supposedly a very bad meal from the low-fat viewpoint. But I felt great during the afternoon after such a lunch. Fats such as butter and cheese can be useful in controlling low blood sugar because they slow down the absorption of carbohydrate.

Many people develop low blood sugar by following the popular high carbohydrate, low-fat diet theories to extreme. They think fruit is a good food and eat lots of it while avoiding foods like eggs, cheese and whole milk. But they could be better off avoiding fruit if they are hypoglycaemic and eating eggs for breakfast.

I believe the best diet for controlling low blood sugar and chronic fatigue syndrome is the good old-fashioned 'balanced diet' with three meals a day. You need to avoid sugar for the first few weeks and then have sweet things occasionally in small amounts as you start feeling better.

Eating snacks can be detrimental if you have a tendency to binge on sweet foods which many people with hypoglycaemia do, in a desperate attempt to make themselves feel better. If you find you can't stop yourself binging on sweet or starchy foods then it's virtually certain that you are suffering from hypoglycaemia. By eating three balanced meals a day, you have the best chance of keeping your blood sugar stable and avoiding destructive sweet snacks.

It takes at least a month to recover from hypoglycaemia by following a balanced diet. Some people start feeling better after a week or two, while others who have been sick a long time might find they need three months or more to start feeling the benefits. Initially, you will almost certainly feel intense cravings for something sweet and may be tempted to lapse. Don't despair. You may have to pick yourself up many times before you can stick to a balanced diet. It just proves that you have been over-dependent on sugar for too long and that you must break the addiction before you can ever expect to enjoy good health again. Keep that as your motivation when the sugar cravings come. Tell yourself: "I might feel bad now, but I'll be ten times worse if I binge".

There were many ups and downs over the next three years as we moved to a new home in the Cotswolds, then to Cardiff where I worked for a magazine publisher. I was well enough to do a day's work and live an almost normal life but I was still not 100 per cent.

I knew diet was crucial to my health but I continued to relapse regularly and eat sweet things or stuff myself with other carbohydrate food, like bread, when I was tired or under stress. Something was still missing from the dietary jigsaw puzzle and I continued to seek until I found it. The answer came unexpectedly in a book I found in a Cardiff bookshop, the name and author of which I cannot now recall. Its message has stuck with me as the cornerstone of my philosophy on diet ever since. It is this: 'Eat when I'm hungry, eat what I'm hungry for, and stop when I've had enough'. It is so simple. But the most profound truths are always the simplest. According to the book we have natural instincts which tell us what to eat, if only we will learn to listen to our bodies. Forget the rules about calories, carbohydrates, fats, vitamins and minerals, and just listen to what your body wants. It will naturally gravitate towards healthy foods. The book also stressed the need to be gentle on yourself when you have a dietary lapse and binge on 'forbidden' food. Don't worry. Just listen to your body and eat less at the next few meals, of simple food, until you get back into balance.

I grasped hold of this new theory and immediately felt a new sense of liberation in the area of diet. I found I could eat small amounts of sweet food, perhaps a muffin or a biscuit, as part of a main meal and not suffer any adverse effects from low blood sugar. Initially I found myself binging on sweet things quite often, as a result of this new, liberated approach to diet and suffered the inevitable ill effects. But I also found I was slowly gaining weight, which I needed to do as I was underweight, and becoming more energetic.

In late 1989 we returned to New Zealand where I worked for a small newspaper in Hokitika and spent one of the most enjoyable years of my life. Then we moved to Ashburton where I spent six years as a reporter at the Ashburton Guardian.

My health and energy gradually improved. There were still bad times, when I got overtired, binged on sweet foods and suffered the inevitable headache and fatigue, but the overall trend was upwards. I started running again and went on several outings of more than twelve kilometres with the local harriers. It was a wonderful feeling to be able to run again. But I found it was easy to overdo it. Often, I pushed myself too far or too fast and came home exhausted. Then I would crave something sweet with the familiar consequences. As many others with chronic fatigue syndrome have discovered, exercise is not the panacea which popular literature portrays it to be. Gentle exercise, yes. But we overdo it at our peril. This has been a hard lesson for me, a former competitive runner, to learn. But painful experience has taught me to listen to my body and to rest when it tells me it is tired.

In September 1996 we moved to Napier, where I spent five years as a journalist with Hawke's Bay Today, one of New Zealand's largest regional daily newspapers. Then I became press secretary for a politician in the New Zealand Parliament in Wellington for two years. These were stressful jobs on top of the demands of a family, but by this time I had learned my limits and how to give my body the right food and rest to ensure good health.

Today, I am a freelance writer and website designer, working from a home-based office in Ashburton. I am 99% recovered from chronic fatigue syndrome. I say 99% rather than 100% because I still sometimes get fatigued more than I would like. I still get headaches when I push myself too hard or eat too much sugar. But I now know the reason. My health is in my hands. It's wonderful to look back and see how far I've come from those dark days twenty years ago.

Most useful aid to recovery - understanding the role that too much sugar can have in my diet and drastically cutting back my sugar consumption.

Recommended books - "I Cured Chronic Fatigue Syndrome - You Can Too" by Jeremy Carew Reid. An inspiring book with a lot of useful information that will help you get well. Based on Ayurvedic principles.

Recommended websites
www.hypoglycemia-diet.com
www.chronicfatigue-help.com
www.newstarget.com : The inside story on Sugar – the real story on sugar and health.

Chris's advice - never lose hope, many others before you have suffered from chronic fatigue syndrome and have come out the other end. Even if it feels now that you will never get well, cling to whatever tiny amount of faith you have. You can get well. You *will* get well. My prayer is that my story will help you on your journey to recovery.

Chris Mole

Katherine's Story

Escaping from a polluted environment saved my life

I succumbed to M.E in the year 2000. Just before the millenium I had been overworking, stressed, not eating properly and exercising whilst tired. I was an accident waiting to happen. In December 1999 I had contracted food poisoning, a virus and a nasty urinary tract infection within the space of a few weeks. I was given antibiotics which made me feel worse and a massive amount of penicillin for a suspected pelvic infection. My immune system collapsed. Within three months I was suffering with chronic fatigue, severe digestive problems, dizziness, brain fog, depression, excruciating burning pains throughout my body, period pain and chemical sensitivities.

I tried hospital after hospital and doctor after doctor, but nobody knew what was wrong with me. I was feeling lonely, angry, vulnerable and scared. I could only just manage a few hours of work a week and consequently acquired a credit card debt. In April 2000 I finally managed to get an appointment with a kinesiologist in London who had an excellent reputation for curing people with chronic fatigue. She immediately diagnosed chronic systemic illness (ME) and prescribed probiotics, anti-fungals, fatty acids and selenium. Within ten days I started to feel better and my recovery began.

Between April 2000 and the summer of 2002 I took a variety of remedies to detoxify and rebuild my immune system, as well as dramatically changing my diet. My practitioner uses the Blood Group Diet. I am Blood Group 0, which meant eliminating wheat, dairy products, oranges and eating plenty of organic meat, fish and vegetables instead. I found this diet to be a tremendous help to my energy levels. I also attended regular yoga classes to assist my nervous system. Counselling was recommended to tackle emotional issues and hyperbaric treatment for ease of symptoms.

Throughout this time I was very lucky to have an extremely supportive man in my life, as well as a close friend who has had ME for nearly eight years. We met through a support group and managed to raise just under £5,000 to enable other sufferers to have free alternative health treatments. We held a nutrition day in January 2003 and this was probably one of the most rewarding days of my life.

In the summer of 2002 my practitioner expressed her concern because I had not made a full recovery. Admittedly I had improved but my chemical sensitivities were still severe and going back to full time work was out of the question. My practitioner wondered if the pollution in the area I was living in was hindering my recovery. In South Essex there is heavy industry along the Estuary as well as masses of traffic and very little countryside. I decided to take a break in Polzeath, North Cornwall where the land is either Royal Duchy organically farmed, or National Trust. Cornwall is the only county without a power station and Polzeath is on the Atlantic Coast. Within a few days of being on holiday I felt less depressed, had more energy and could breathe more easily. I returned home to Essex after just one week in Polzeath and within twenty-four hours felt terrible. My breathing was laboured, my chemical sensitivities soared and I couldn't stop crying. All I could smell were car fumes. I told my friends and family that I had to move and in September 2002 I settled in North Cornwall. Within a few weeks my depression had gone, I had more energy, I was sleeping better, my period pain had improved and my chemical sensitivities were ameliorated.

Subsequently I decided to go back to work full-time. I started helping my partner with his theatre company and also thought about running my own business. In May 2003 I bought a beautiful big house in Chapel Amble, not far from Polzeath, and decided to open an organic, chemical free B&B suitable for people with allergies, ME or Multiple Chemical Syndrome, and this is proving to be a real success. Moving to Cornwall was the most influential part of my recovery. It is a beautiful place to live and work. Moving to a cleaner area might not work for everyone with ME but escaping from a polluted environment has literally saved my life.

I now walk six miles around the coast of Cornwall and socialise with friends without feeling ill afterwards! I enjoy reading books again, I swim in the sea throughout the summer months and I love going to the theatre and seeing films.

Now I am living life to the full!

Most useful aid to recovery - moving to a healthier environment

Recommended website - www.afme.org.uk

Katherine's advice - my advice is to join support groups, contact Action for ME, eat organic food, stop using chemicals on yourself and in your home, do as much of your own research as you can, don't rely on the National Health Service to get you well and don't give up hope!

Katherine Austen

Matt's Story

Kettlebell exercises are a lot of fun

My energy took a downward course one Sunday afternoon in November 2000 - five months before I finally ground to a halt. That afternoon I was hung over and a bit slow on the uptake when I answered my front door to an irate middle- aged man. He was convinced someone was spying on him and convinced that that someone was me. He had a bit of a rant, most of which I didn't understand and then he started punching me. The first two punches were just taps on the chin, the third a heavy roundhouse punch that broke the jaw in two places and shattered a wisdom tooth. Reason obviously wasn't going to get me far in this situation so I backed away and apologised, which meant he could leave satisfied he had dealt with a threat to his privacy and I got someone with an obvious drug or psychiatric problem out of my house.

Three days later I left hospital with a Titanium plate holding my jaw together, looking like someone making an attempt on the record for sucking the world's largest gobstopper. I thought it would probably take a few weeks for me to feel like myself again. But it took years, not weeks.

During winter life became more difficult. I just managed to squeeze out the energy to get me to work every day but everything was a strain. Light and noise seemed to get more intense and more wearing. Every day tasks became minor stresses and minor stresses became major ones. Worst of all I had a permanent headache and felt dizzy much of the time. I carried on working but planned a couple of weeks holiday in the Spring so there was something to look forward to. My energy kept on dropping; not only was I tired but I was acutely stressed, with nerves often tingling and burning, so I felt constantly on edge. Although the symptoms were different, I took St John's Wort for mild winter depression, which had worked before.

Over Christmas and New Year the office was closed giving me a ten-day break which I hoped would enable me to rest properly and sort my energies out. But when the New Year began my energy was still dropping and stress levels intensifying.

In February a friend suggested going to a cranial osteopath for the dizziness. I went along and my initial reaction was that I had wasted my money, because the osteopath was holding my head and apparently not doing anything, unlike a massage or acupressure session. In actual fact that session probably prevented me doing more lasting damage to myself, as I immediately began getting the sleep my body really needed.

In early March I went for a walk with my father across the Clifton Downs, an area of open ground in Bristol on the cliffs above the Avon Gorge. As we walked back to the house against a bitter March wind the effort of putting one foot in front of the other began to seem unbearable. As I panted for breath I faced up to the fact that for a supposedly fit thirty year old who walked everywhere the fifteen minute walk home would probably destroy me. I had my mobile so my mother soon picked us up and drove us home in quiet and I spent the rest of the day in bed. The next day my doctor signed me off work, advised me to rest and then to just wait and see. He diagnosed a delayed shock reaction from the assault, which fitted the progress of my illness. When pressed she reckoned six months of recovery as a maximum. I was very lucky to have her as my GP. Throughout my illness she always made time for me, gave me the benefit of her professional experience, but equally allowed me to make my own judgements about dealing with my illness.

Cranial osteopathy helped both in reducing my headaches and my sleep from sixteen hours a night to ten. I had acupuncture and Chinese herbal medicine to boost my basic store of energy. I knew that I had driven myself into a deep level of exhaustion through sheer willpower as I had attempted to carry on, so I was deep in energy debt. I thought at least two or three months full time rest would be required. I resigned from my job.

The most pronounced symptoms seemed to come from the site of the original injury. Low down on my left jaw I had a titanium plate, close to the nerve which runs down to the chin. This frequently felt cold or numb as my surgeon had warned me it would. What was less expected was that any contact with this plate opened a sluice gate for the very worst of my symptoms. Any kind of massage, no matter how gentle or how brief would trigger off a reaction in the nerves and muscles surrounding the injury, usually a few hours later or the next day.

Instead of recovering, my exhaustion was apparently digging deeper. I will never forget standing in the garden one morning, feeling as though a steel vice was being tightened on either side of my head. With another slight turn of the thread my head would implode on itself. I could barely speak or move as my entire consciousness had become that unrelenting point of pain, and that was the only time I considered suicide during my illness. If those experiences were to be part of my daily life I decided I would be entirely justified in ending it some months down the line. But luckily with time and the cranial osteopathy, the pain eased off enough to be just bearable and I learned how to avoid the worst of the headaches. That morning will forever reside in my memory as probably the worst moment of my life.

In the October of that first year I relapsed, barely able to stay awake for more than four hours a day for a while and in light of that, my doctor diagnosed Chronic Fatigue Syndrome. Like most people I did my research on the illness. Books on ME/CFS mostly concluded that any treatments were either ineffective or would at best alleviate your symptoms only slightly. The basic message was you are stuck with this illness until it runs out of steam or reaches a level of stability where you can live a part-time life, a bit of work and socialising, but lots of rest, frustration and unfulfilled potential.

There were ME support groups available of course but I had no interest in them - the last thing I wanted to do was sit in a room full of sickly people telling each other how ill they feel, the cumulative effect of so much ill health eroding everyone's energy and more importantly, their hope. Maybe I wrote them off unnecessarily. Perhaps some of these groups had a more positive tone than I imagined, but with limited energy any trip to a public place would be exhausting and stressful, so I wasn't inclined to take the chance.

Having hit several low points and knowing I was in for the long haul I kept a very careful watch on my symptoms with an A5 diary of any exercises or treatments so I could establish ground rules of how to look after myself. I didn't know exactly why I was feeling so ill but I was never in any doubt that my symptoms were very real and very physical. The diary was invaluable because my body rarely reacted immediately to circumstances. If, out of frustration, I went for a longer walk than usual, I would not feel the effects straight away, instead it would be the next day or some days later.

Qi Qong in small doses gave me a little extra energy and luckily from years of Qi Qong practice I had a store of specific exercises to deal with specific symptoms.

About a year and a half in I read an interesting article in the paper about an old fashioned form of weight training called kettlebells. They go back to the ancient Greeks and were largely forgotten about in the West during the twentieth century. But Russian athletes trained with kettlebells and that was one of the reasons for Russian dominance of the Olympics during the post war period. Kettlebell weights are little more than cannonballs with a handle on the top, like an old fashioned kettle that sits on a stove. There are various ways to use them, but essentially because the weight pivots on the end of the handle it is more like swinging a weight than lifting it and this means you must employ the core muscles around your middle and in your spine to support the movement in your arms.

My legs seemed to get disproportionately tired with ME, even a short walk could leave them hot and burning. I really wanted to get back to some form of exercise but needed something that didn't place an emphasis on the leg muscles. I thought of kettlebells - they seemed like a better way of doing things than all the complicated equipment which makes up the modern gym. I started with a homemade weight of 5kg to see how my energy would respond and even after only a few days it led to some definite improvement.

Strangely enough the intensity of kettlebell training in a short burst seemed to be better than a longer period of more gentle exercise like Qi Qong. Suddenly my walks became comfortable at thirty minutes instead of a previous maximum of twenty. I felt less on edge and my sleeping patterns improved. Where I think they helped me was that they develop strong muscles around the spine, helping the spine to support itself and take pressure off both the sympathetic and parasympathetic nervous systems. This meant the nerves could relax properly and so more energy became available.

Kettlebell exercises are a lot of fun and are an amazing form of exercise because they very quickly take you to your physical limits. Say for example you're doing twenty repetitions, the first ten will probably feel quite comfortable. But suddenly, maybe after the twelfth, your lungs start hurting, your muscles go heavy and completing the set becomes a real chore; each repetition not just increasing but apparently multiplying the workload. Around repetition fifteen or sixteen you're thinking you'll never make it and the only way through is to concentrate on getting one closer to your goal. Somehow you get to number twenty, drop the weight, sink to your knees and gasp for breath. Take a drink of water, give yourself a minute and then pick up the weight and do same number with the other arm. I found I could do this incredibly taxing exercise and strangely my energy was increasing. Most importantly, while I may have felt exhausted immediately after exercising, in the following days I would have *more* energy - the opposite of how I seemed to respond with nearly all other exercise with ME/CFS.

This gave me real hope of recovering and it became easier to think ahead and beyond this illness. One of the great difficulties of ME is what to do with all the time available. More time than energy is a recipe for boredom. As most people with ME find public places especially wearing you need to occupy a great deal of time on your own. I managed to accomplish quite a lot in my time ill.

I started by buying a good digital piano and a CD Rom so I could finally learn to read music. This worked pretty well because the program can tell you exactly what you're doing wrong and set exercises to correct your weak points. Eventually I found a piano teacher, precisely eight minutes walk away and downhill on the way home, so I knew even if the lesson was tiring I would always make it back.

My days were not so bad if the headaches and stress levels were at low levels. I developed an appreciation of classical music thanks to Radio 3, having the time to listen to whole concertos and symphonies. There were always good black and white films to watch in the afternoons. In the summer times I watched the cricket coverage and was able to learn the subtleties of the game from Channel 4's coverage at a time when the English cricket team had finally learned to win matches. I also started a website for people with ME to pass on all the exercises and treatments that had given me some improvement, particularly the osteopathy and the kettlebells. Of course I was still tired and stressed for no reason, but at my parents' comfortable suburban house, with large garden and two cats, a good day was reasonably pleasant, particularly as I had started to believe I would get better - even if life was being experienced through a consciousness permanently shrouded in fog.

My career in IT had been put on hold for the moment but I signed up for home study courses with the Open University, leading to an undergraduate Diploma in Computing. I was able to work at home, pacing myself and working when I had the energy. Most importantly at no extra cost they would send an invigilator so I could sit the exams at home, preserving my limited energies and giving me the best possible chance of getting a decent grade.

Living with ME at any level means a degree of isolation. I was disappointed that I lost contact with most of my friends. It would have been so much harder to keep going without my parents, who were superb. They did everything they could to help from the practical support of giving lifts, shopping, cooking and putting up with having a constantly tired sickly person in their home twenty-four hours a day without any respite. But of course they were also able to hear my frustrations and they knew when to step in with an offer of help and when to just leave me to it. They were more than my parents. Throughout this time they were my best friends and I am eternally grateful for having them to stand by me.

I joined an internet dating site, not exactly expecting to find the love of my life but thinking I could at least sharpen up my social skills via the keyboard. I met a nurse who only lived two streets away. We met in a cafe at a very manageable ten minutes walk and got on well. Luckily she wasn't expecting us to go white water rafting every weekend and most of her nights out meant a trip to the local pub. Ideal for me with my condition. So it seemed after two and a half years I would finally have a girlfriend.

But of course it wasn't that simple. My weight training had given me more energy but public places were still hard work and the difference between doing something when I was ready for it and keeping to other people's schedules was immense. I had become better at managing public places over that year but only because I could choose when to make these trips - when my energy was good. It wasn't so easy with my girlfriend. I would arrange to meet her but often have to cancel at the last minute. Soon it became apparent that no matter how understanding she was, I could not be myself and we could not have a relationship. After three weeks we called it a day which made 2003 a particularly miserable Christmas. That long period of re-runs on TV was spent reflecting that not only was part-time work still out of the question, but also that by some run of fate I had met a beautiful, intelligent, kind hearted woman I was beginning to care deeply about and this damn illness had just slapped down any hope of my having a relationship with her.

The 2003/2004 winter was probably one of the most testing psychologically. I had come so far and worked so hard to get myself better and yet my body was still reacting badly to changes in routine and any meaningful attempts to move my life on. I had a feeling that there was very little I could control about my life. I started meditating at least twenty minutes every day, which would at least keep my mind from analysing my situation over and over. And occasionally meditation just clears the mind enough to help you to find the answers.

In February 2004 I contacted Jennie, a friend who I had shared a house with many years ago in Ireland. I sent her an email bringing her up to date on my situation and how it was getting to me. The reply came back, "Hey that thing you've got, CFS. Is that the same as ME? Because I know someone who cures it!"

The treatment was named Reverse Therapy. The Reverse Therapy view is that ME is actually the product of an over-active hypothalamus. The body/mind believes we are under threat and goes into overdrive trying to alert us to take action in response. So the ME head fog occurs because the brain is being set up for action not thought; sore muscles are constantly being primed for activity and glands swell as the immune system prepares to defend us from non-existent bugs. Unsurprisingly in time the result of all this is total exhaustion. To resolve this the client and therapist work out a message which represents what the body and mind are concerned about. This is written on a card and whenever symptoms increase the client goes to a quiet place, reads the card, then takes some sort of action which demonstrates to the body and mind that the problem has been addressed. With the problem resolved the hypothalamus is free to switch off the symptoms of ME and allow the body to function normally. Even the length and severity of the illness should not affect chances of success - for some people the alarms may be sounding louder and longer - but once the switch has been flipped the result should be the same, no more symptoms.

In the second session the therapist saw links with the lead in to my illness. As I explained to the therapist, in the year leading up to my illness it seemed peoples' perception of me was often at odds with my perception of myself. In short my boss had treated me as if I were an idiot and all the women I met just seemed to want one night stands, with no hope of a relationship. This happens to everyone of course and on it's own it wasn't going to bring about ME. What it took was a random violent assault by a total stranger who was convinced I was spying on him. This in the most dramatic and immediate way was telling my hypothalamus that there was a huge gulf between my external and internal worlds! Most significantly because the assault was so quick and unexpected I had not *reacted* - I had failed to get my arms up to defend myself or fight back. Sure I had later decided it was probably safer to move from that house, but that was some weeks after and the lack of an immediate response was taken by the hypothalamus as a signal that I wasn't doing anything about this problem.

The whole process of Reverse Therapy usually takes several sessions as it's not always obvious what these messages are. Clients may get a new message in each session, or a refinement of an existing message. In my six months of treatment I had four messages, one of which I felt was really too general, but the others did seem to generate a definite response. In fact there was nothing magical about these messages per se. Instead they were just keys to open a dialogue with my body-mind. What matters was that I responded to these symptoms so that the body-mind and hypothalamus got some feedback, which showed I was dealing with the problem.

So did it work for me? Yes no doubt. By January 2005 I began working again full time. In June 2005 I went to Andalusia in Spain by myself, wandering about in temperatures over 100 degrees, then came back to a front row seat watching the England cricket team beating Australia in my home town, before starting a new job the next day - all within the space of two weeks. Heat, noise, crowds, strange cities, offices - none of this would have been possible a year before. Most importantly I was aware that I had lost over three years of my life and my first priority was to get on with living what I've got left, because time is a luxury in short supply.

Thankfully I now have my health and an understanding of what made me ill and how to prevent it happening again. So I should never again have to calculate if I will be able to get to the end of my street to post a letter or have enough energy remaining for the two minute walk home.

Most useful aid to recovery - Reverse Therapy

Matthew Benton

Howard's Story

Reflections of an ex-chronic fatigue sufferer

Between May and November 1994 I had a series of three hepatitis B vaccinations due to work place risks. Although I can't prove it, nor would most medical professionals support the idea, I have no doubt that this was a trigger. In talking with other CFS sufferers, many had a vaccination or vaccinations in the months leading up to the initial onset of their condition or they had a major relapse after a vaccination.

Easter time 1995 I came down with a viral illness, which put me in bed for about eight days. A full series of blood tests could only tell me what I did not have. My energy and stamina never fully recovered after that illness, although at the time it didn't really occur to me. Initially, I though I was just getting old – at twenty-nine! Slowly, my lack of energy became frustratingly worse.

In July 1997 chicken pox put me in bed for about ten days. My digestive system never completely recovered and irritable bowel syndrome set in. At the time I was on holiday but chose to resign from work mainly due to my health. I had struggled to do some part time work for three months but had to give it up in April 1998 because I wasn't coping. During this time several very stressful events took place in my life, including the birth of our first child in September 1995, who was eventually diagnosed with a rare, degenerative, genetic, muscle and brain disorder. Without a doubt, this long-term stressful environment was another trigger for my susceptibility to CFS.

Going along to the local CFS support group for the first three to four times was very informative and encouraging. I was glad to discover I wasn't the only person struggling to find an understanding doctor who was prepared to do anything after endless rounds of blood tests didn't reveal anything significantly wrong. It was also good to find a comprehensive lending library of very informative books, tapes and videos. Depressing though many of the discoveries I made were, there is still a real liberation in understanding exactly what you are dealing with. Taking away the fear of the unknown in the early visits to the support group lifted a huge emotional burden off me. It gave me more resources to cope with the strange symptoms I was struggling with ...

... which included in basic order of severity of debility – fatigue and weakness, breathing was a real effort some days, light headedness and dizziness, muscle pain (fibromyalgia) especially in the upper legs; fairly constant headaches, joint pain especially in the ankles, wrists and fingers, inability to sleep or unrefreshing sleep, night sweats, sore throat or ears, churning painful stomach and associated diarrhoea especially at night; hot flushed face feeling, itchy gritty eyes, sweaty feeling around the eyes, cold sore feet, no matter what the temperature of the day or how much I covered them up, 'brain fog',confusion, poor short term memory ..... and so on!

For a long time, I felt that I could beat this condition if I followed a very strict healthy diet avoiding the five 'whites' of salt, sugar, dairy products, white flour products and all animal fats and products, aiming for an 80% raw fruit and vegetable diet while drinking plenty of clean water and vegetable juices, in particular carrot juice. Dietary changes did initially help – getting off dairy products particularly as tests later revealed that I was lactose intolerant - but the improvement was not sustained and I became obsessive about what I did or didn't put in my mouth, which was counter-productive. While very important, diet was not the source of my healing.

I also tried many different and often expensive vitamins, minerals, supplements, natural remedies and so on, with no significant improvements. I got to the stage where I refused to try a new product unless I heard first hand from another CFS sufferer that they had gained sustained improvement from it.

As the weeks rolled into months and then years I found going along to the support group frustrating and depressing. Sharing with others, all struggling with similar aches and pains and no real solutions was *not* helping me. I needed to become part of a support group with people who had *recovered* from the condition. Those people seemed few and far between, which is a depressing statement in itself, and a reflection of the nature of the condition. Generally, people who had recovered were out living life and wanted to put space between themselves and CFS.

I now find myself an ex-CFS sufferer. *Praise God!* I have known the fear of being curled up in a foetal position in bed all day, with intense muscle pain from head to toe and the strongest dose of painkiller in the house only just taking the edge off it. Sitting still in a cold bath of water for ten minutes several times a day did provide some relief to the intense muscle pain. (Extraction of wisdom teeth is the only worse pain I have experienced. However, it was localized to my head, and I knew it would end when the gum healed). I have known the strain on our marriage as my wife struggled with the frustration of having to cuddle up to a slimy, sweaty husband for months, who was often too weak to even return a decent hug.

My heartfelt desire in sharing the story of how I was released from CFS is that it may assist others to find a pathway of healing from this debilitating illness. I have no desire to be controversial, but must share the truth of how God set me free.

On Saturday the 5th of June 1999 I attended a seminar on the cults/occult and in particular, Freemasonry. At the end of that night there was a time of corporate prayer, out loud, specifically renouncing the generational curses that come about as a result of the oaths taken in Masonic rituals. I have never been a Mason and have rejected becoming involved, however, I understand at least three generations of my forefathers have been Masons. At the end of that night God through his Holy Spirit did some major surgery in my life. Since that night all the major symptoms of CFS in my body have ceased!

For a day or two after that night, I had a deep healing pain in my bones, interestingly one of the main sources of the immune system. Two days later, I went on a four day break with my wife which had been planned months before, during which we walked four to five kilometres per day. I had rarely walked with my wife for years before that, and would have to turn back early if I did. I had to be careful and not over-do things for a while, as I still sometimes struggled with tiredness and my muscles were occasionally sore and stiff due to the shock of extra use and after years of inactivity. I still occasionally struggled with digestive problems, but this has now normalized.

In over seven years since that night, I have had one relapse when all the symptoms of CFS returned for two days in bed, from which I received release by prayerfully renouncing Masonic curses in a similar way to the night of my original healing.

My stamina and energy levels have now returned to pre-1995 levels. Having been largely removed from society for nearly three years, I had some emotional struggles in the area of confidence to overcome. Since my healing I have remained the primary care giver for my profoundly disabled son, completed a four year university education degree and currently work as a high school chaplain.

Over the years of sharing my journey of healing with others, either face to face or over the Internet, I have often come across people expressing the view that once you have had CFS you always have it, and even though you may recover from it you will relapse again within five years. It is so refreshing to be free of living with the emotional pressure in fear of this being the case for me. This is particularly so in view of the high care needs of my son.

I have vivid memories of having to crawl across our living room floor one day to ring a neighbour to come and help me change the nappies of both my boys because I had crashed out on the floor while my wife was out working to try and keep the household financially afloat. As demanding a task as it is to care for my son, I am forever grateful that I now have the health to do so and the energy to enjoy regular wrestling matches with his very healthy brother on the same floor that I found myself crawling across or lying on in the darkest days of my battle with CFS!

Through the hardest months of my illness, I declared I would widely promote and sell anything that gave me sustained release from CFS. I promote to you the healing power of Jesus Christ, through the renouncing of generational curses. I can't sell it to you however, because it will not cost you anything!

Most useful aid to recovery - the healing power of Jesus Christ

Recommended websites
www.jubilee.org.nz
www.sozo.org
www.cwlinc.com
www.hodderheadline.co.uk/index.asp?url=bookdetails.
asp&book=457&best
www.hacres.com
www.sa.democrats.org.au/parlt/budget99/0803_e.htm

Howard's advice - my challenge to you is to prayerfully consider your spiritual heritage and seek out people and resources to assist you with any issues, which may be keeping you in ill health. By all means continue to pursue all possible issues that may be causing your illness, but don't spend lots of money and time pursuing others while ignoring/neglecting the spiritual. If in many cases CFS is spiritually rooted, we should not find it surprising that medical science is finding the mysteries of the illness hard to unravel, by the testing of physical body specimens.

Howard

Christine's Story

I have become a parrot boarding house

At last I can legitimately bore someone with the history of my ME. I don't go into it among friends, in case their eyes glaze over – although I must say I have had great support and understanding from them and my family. People I haven't seen for a while are amazed that I am so well, especially that I can walk for miles again like I did before. As I don't drive, it's always been my main mode of transport.

I think perhaps the main reason my doctor was so sympathetic and as good as diagnosed my illness herself, was because it was a direct result of a viral illness from which I never fully recovered. So a reason for it could be seen. People who become gradually ill over a long period, perhaps due to stress, don't have such an obvious cause, and if they're unlucky their doctor is less likely to say it's ME and more inclined to say it's depression. Maybe because I didn't become depressed, I recovered my physical health more than some do, because I was always planning what I would do tomorrow/next week/next month and so on.

For the first two or three years, I fought against it, really believing I could overcome it by deciding to do something and doing it. So not being able to do it made me angry and more determined to do it tomorrow. It could be washing my hair, reading a magazine or being taken out for example. I always accepted invitations, then felt terrible about having to decline at the last minute – as if I was letting people down. Then one day, having read somewhere that you should accept your illness and its limitations and stop fighting it, I did just that. I stopped planning and then fretting at failing and from then on also felt less angry. All this time I was actually sleeping most of the day – and unfortunately, *not* most of the night; the short spaces between sleeps were spent relaxing and going with the flow, and only trying to do something if I really felt I wanted to, not because I felt I ought to.

After I had been ill about five years I was still sleeping a lot, feeling most of the time on the verge of fainting (I never did) and walking, on good days, and in slow motion, the length of the garden or out to the car. We moved house at this time and it was very difficult. Looking back I wonder how we got through it. Everybody said they thought I'd get better in the country air, surrounded by trees and fields. I don't think it made any difference at all. It was hard work and for a while I was worse. But gradually I spent less time needing to sleep. I slept only in the afternoons – not the mornings and evenings too! I was able to do a bit of artwork sometimes and I joined the ME writer's circle and did a bit of writing, but I always felt very ill after only half-an-hour.

As my original illness, pleurisy, affected my chest and breathing, it was always these symptoms that returned when I over-stretched myself. I never had any digestive problems or headaches. It was always the chest and legs.

I think my natural optimistic tendency kept me from becoming depressed (fed-up, yes!) and that in itself I believe, made me want to do things and increased my physical capabilities. I also had to look after my parrots, and as my middle son Joe said, "it's having them to see to that makes you get up in the morning". Of course, as soon as I'd cleaned and fed them, I had to go and lie down again. I had quite a lot in aviaries when I became ill, and most had to go. I still have some and since moving to the country and getting better I have become a 'parrot boarding house'.

I also wrote and illustrated a 'diary' for "Parrots" magazine for a couple of years, going from a couple of paragraphs to a double page spread. That came to an end when a new editor took over and stopped all the regular articles and started a fresh lot. However, I am on the 'helpline' of the magazine and get quite a lot of phone calls from panicking parrot owners.

I'm now doing a lot of art and craft work. I belong to two art clubs – one of which I started - and work at my local country market on Friday mornings where I sell things I make and am in charge of the kitchen. I suppose this means that I am in effect back at work, and if I was not past retirement age I could have gone back, but it wasn't until I reached sixty nearly four years ago that I could say I was well enough to do so – by which time it was too late!

I do think that having several totally absorbing interests were what helped me recover. If my whole life had revolved around my job (part-time teaching crafts to adults), then not being able to do that would have been devastating, and I think this is what makes some people depressed, particularly as one's social life is often involved with one's work colleagues. Mine wasn't, so I didn't have that to lose. My social life has always revolved around my art and parrots (I ran the Bristol branch of the Parrot Society until I became ill) and that was easy to gradually pick up again as I got better.

Because I wasn't prescribed any medication (I just took painkillers when my thighs were really bad), I can't ascribe my recovery to anything but luck and allowing the illness to run its course.

I couldn't afford to try any alternative methods or therapies, though several were suggested to me. I didn't want to as I didn't really think they would help. Many seemed to involve diet, assuming you had problems in that area, which I didn't, or exercise, which I was horrified at the prospect of, knowing that any physical or mental exercise made me worse. I felt I was already moving around as much as I could and knew how far I could push myself, without some physiotherapist telling me what to do. In effect I governed my illness myself I suppose and that seems to have worked for me. Actually, I'm just remembering something I did try, but not really of my own volition.

It was before we moved and I decided to join the ME watercolour group, run by a woman who was a non-practicing (due to ME) homeopath. The group was in the morning because all of us needed to sleep in the afternoons. I was really keen to meet new people, but in fact gave up after two or three weeks because it made me feel too ill.

The homeopath said that she thought she could give me something, free of charge, that would perhaps help me. I was intrigued because I was so disappointed that a quiet hour and a half of painting was making me so exhausted. I asked her what it was but she said I didn't need to know and would tell me after I'd taken it for a week, when we would know if it had had any effect.

So I went home with seven mini-pills wrapped in tissue and took one a day. The effect was immediate. I became hyperactive, almost manic. Derek confessed afterwards that he was seriously concerned. I couldn't stop talking and most amazingly I was dashing about at full speed, to the shops, to friends, then collapsing in the evenings exhausted, but not being able to sleep. I was up in the night, writing and painting. No wonder Derek and Joe were worried. After four or five days I stopped taking them and soon became normal again – normal as before I took them, not normal before ME!

It was wonderful being so active, but I think it did more harm than good, as I soon felt worse than I had done before the tablets. I was too poorly to go to the next painting session and when I finally did and told my new friend how I'd been, she was very sorry. She said you never can be sure how much of something anyone should take because everyone is so different. I said perhaps I could have half the dose she'd given me and that would make me feel just right, but she said no, it was too risky, and I mustn't have anymore.

I then persuaded her to tell me what this 'magic' potion was. So she did. It was snake venom! I then realised why she wouldn't tell me before I took it! What I couldn't understand was how my legs, which alternated between feeling like jelly or lead when trying to walk, and ached and throbbed when at rest, suddenly became normal and could walk – fast. It really was like magic.

I now regard myself as 99.9% cured. I can lead a normal life. Just occasionally I get the painful thighs and chest, though not very severe and more a little warning that perhaps I've been doing too much. This happens no more than once every few weeks. The other legacy of my illness and inactivity is that I put on weight and I am still trying to get it off, which is very annoying. Having always been slim and now being active again and always having eaten a healthy diet, it's taking a long time to lose that weight.

I hope that all this rambling has been of some interest and of use to anyone with ME that might read it.

Most useful aid to recovery - peace and quiet and someone to look after you

Recommended book - thirteen years ago there were no books. The ME Association newsletter was useful.

Christine's advice - don't fight it, go with it

Christine Goodall

Clare's Story

Beyond the Glass Cage

"I live in a glass cage - the invisible walls around me are impenetrable. Beyond them lies a barrage of symptoms. Illness cost me my job, my social life, my role in the family, my access to activity and my ability to rely on my body to function predictably."

I wrote those words eight years ago. I was virtually bedridden for eighteen months, used a wheelchair to go out and appeared in my dreams as disabled. Now I have totally recovered. For the past ten years I have made no concessions at all to ME. Like anyone, I have boundaries to my resources and well-being. The difference now is that I bounce back rapidly every time; my body can restore its balance. Here is my story - a streamlined account of a stumbling journey.

I see my recovery from ME as similar to healing a cut finger. My body has an inborn ability to repair itself. I can't force healing to happen, but I can affect it. If I fail to clean the cut or I pick at the scab, if I have poor circulation, work in a cold environment or have a deficient diet - all these hinder the healing process. I can encourage healing by dressing and protecting the wound. Before my illness I was a doctor (GP) and some of my symptoms, sore throat, swollen glands and flu-like malaise, strongly suggested an on-going infection. With no medical cure available, all I could do was help my body to help itself.

There were four cornerstones to my recovery. Wholeness - I learned to use body, mind and spirit together to unlock one another, instead of keeping each in separate boxes. Change - ME unhinged my familiar circumstances and relationships, opening me to explore deeper areas of mindsets and habits. Balance - I discovered the importance of allowing opposites each to have their own place in my life. Love - I experienced the reality of the bible verse, 'I healed them … with cords of human kindness, with ties of love.' (Hosea ch11v4)

These are the things I tried, starting with the most helpful. A combined body/mind/spirit approach; accepting help from family, friends and professionals; Pacing - developing a sustainable daily pattern; finding hope, love and meaning in my circumstances, helped by faith and prayer; developing balance in as many areas of my life as possible; nutritional supplements including Efamol; anti-depressants to treat a brief spell of depression; charting progress to keep me objective and homeopathy.

Recovery began with the hardest part of all, facing the truth of the existence and severity of my illness and disability. This set me free to begin the journey of recovery from a place that was real, and therefore solid to build on. It gave me the opportunity to fight with the illness rather than fighting against it. No more imagining I would be better tomorrow. No more trying to live beyond my resources. I was face to face with the pain of all I had lost. Grief is a minefield of emotion - anger, frustration, sadness, longing, loneliness, fear, guilt, worthlessness, self-pity and despair. I needed to acknowledge and defuse these feelings in order to avoid becoming disabled by them.

Learning how to budget my meagre energy was essential. However, as I struggled to balance activity and rest I encountered other imbalances. Keeping busy was as instinctive to me as breathing but I was uncomfortable with stillness; change was invigorating though I hated routine; I enjoyed helping people, while independence and pride made receiving difficult. The key was to develop those qualities which I had previously lacked, to establish balance throughout my life.

I worked out a pattern of activity and rest which I could sustain even on a bad day, so my body knew what to expect and prepare for and I didn't squander energy fretting about meeting the needs of the day.

Accepting help, compromising, delegating and saying no were essential, but difficult. I spent my energy firstly on what mattered most to me - nurturing the people who nurtured me, especially my husband, Ian, and our young sons. Ian needed encouragement in his role as carer, and I needed his support to keep me going. We enlisted help from different people for as many tasks as possible, trying not to be unrealistic in our expectations but to ask only for the what that individual could best give. Slowly, in fits and starts, I drew more into my periods of activity. I could cope with the routine and discipline as long as I allowed space for fun, creativity and mistakes - of which I made plenty.

I learned relaxation skills to improve the quality of my rest times. As I relaxed physically I began to listen to what was happening inside me. I encountered the emotions I listed above and realised how much of my precious energy was being squandered on such baggage. Counselling helped me to start unpacking.

In tandem with this I began searching the Christian faith, at the heart of which is love. Exploring my relationship with God shed light on my relationships both with others and with myself. I had been taught, 'Love your neighbour as yourself', but the implied 'love yourself as your neighbour' had never occurred to me. The experience of being valued for who I am, not for what I do, freed me to acknowledge my own needs and set out to address them. This was primarily a spiritual journey, but it unlocked the physical dimension as well.

Instead of ignoring my body I began to *listen* carefully to it and heed warning signals. I took advice about nutrition and vitamin supplements, avoided large or irregular meals and excluded foods which my body couldn't easily handle. Anti-depressants countered a brief spell of depression (though they had no effect on my original symptoms) and I tried Efamol and homeopathy.

One day something amazing happened. For the first time in over three years I woke up without a sore throat, and my swollen glands soon disappeared. I was able to become physically tired again - previously flu-like malaise had stopped me reaching that stage. Somehow my body had gathered enough resources to throw off whatever infection I had been harbouring.

The journey back to full health plus sufficient energy reserves took almost three more years. Six years in all. Step by step, I reclaimed roles, relationships and responsibilities. It was a bit like growing up all over again, moving from dependence and vulnerability towards independence and responsibility. There were fears to overcome as I moved from the familiar and secure towards the uncertain. Whenever I tried to gain ground too fast I relapsed, undermining my confidence.

In the end, with help and support, I got there. Life is not the same as it was beforehand, because I choose to spend my time and energy differently, in a healthier and more balanced way. I prefer my new life and wouldn't swap back to what I had before. Nor would I ever wish to re-enter the living nightmare that is ME. Yet both my husband, Ian, and I, feel that our family has in the long run gained more than we lost. We found unexpected treasures in those dark days. One of the most powerful things ME taught me is that I can choose to change. I needn't fear my weaknesses or my feelings: they are windows of opportunity, inviting me towards a wholeness that goes beyond my physical recovery.

"Bon voyage" for your own journey.

1. Fleming, C. The Glass Cage, British Medical Journal 19 March 1994 Vol 308, p797.

Most useful aids to recovery - Hope that recovery is possible. People who believed in me and supported me. A desire to learn and to change the things that needed changing, to accept the things I could not change and to search for the wisdom to know the difference.

Recommended websites
www.afme.org.uk
www.drmyhill.co.uk

Dr. Clare Fleming

Fiona's story

A stretch in time

In 1989 I was running a successful public relations company. My job was very stressful and I worked long hours with no time for lunch breaks or holidays. To prop up my flagging energy levels I ate lots of junk food and sweet things. Then when I went home I would drink a bottle of wine to numb the exhaustion and slow down my racing brain, heating up a ready-prepared meal in the microwave.

The first warning that all was not well was the panic attacks. For no apparent reason I would start to feel shaky, anxious and strange, and have difficulty getting my breath. This was followed by chronic insomnia, sometimes going for two or three nights without sleeping at all. Still I ignored the distress signals my body was sending me and the fact that I was becoming incredibly fatigued, and I worked even harder. I also started squeezing an aerobics class into my lunch hour. In fact, I didn't really think about the fatigue, I assumed that life was like that and it was something I just had to accept.

Then I got what I thought was flu. After three days in bed I dragged myself back to work. Despite feeling wiped out and dizzy, I thought I had to work or my world would cave in – especially as I owed the bank £50,000 on my business account and had a huge mortgage. My doctor took some blood tests and later told me I had glandular fever caused by the Epstein-Barr virus. She advised me to rest, so I slowed down a bit

- but not enough. Three months later I sold my business and started working as a television researcher, but soon developed some unnerving symptoms that I couldn't ignore. The exhaustion would get so bad that sometimes I couldn't speak, and would have to go and lie down. One day my husband found me on the floor – I couldn't move. Even after resting I was still tired. Nonetheless I managed to struggle on with my job, lying down during my lunch hour rather than socialising with others in the production team. I managed to keep my condition secret from colleagues. To admit to being exhausted or ill wasn't allowed in our driven work environment.

Ultimately I became so ill that I had to give up work. Resting didn't make me any better and if I exercised it took me days to recover. My muscles ached, I had a permanent fog in my head and I couldn't sleep. Eventually I was diagnosed with M.E. or chronic fatigue syndrome. If only I had listened to my body when it had first sent me signals to slow down.

My health deteriorated until in 1992 I was in a wheelchair for six months. At this point I was too tired even to hold a conversation. I was also facing increasing prejudice from some of my friends and family, misled by inaccurate media coverage of ME, while many doctors were very scathing and didn't believe that I had a genuine physical illness.

In the end I was taken into the Priory hospital in Kent for three months, paid for by my health insurance. There I was put on various drugs including MAOI anti-depressants which, in hindsight, made me much worse. However I was also taught how to meditate and given cognitive behaviour therapy by a wonderful therapist who totally accepted the physical nature of my illness. CBT didn't improve my energy but it did make me feel more hopeful about my life and the future.

In 1993 local yoga teacher Angela Stevens asked if I would help her set up a special class for people with ME/CFS. She'd noticed that this illness was on the increase and thought that remedial yoga might help. I wasn't so sure – strenuous exercise was the last thing I needed

– but Angela assured me that gentle yoga would be beneficial. So I got together a group of people and we gave it a go.

Almost immediately I began to feel better. Angela concentrated on yoga breathing, relaxation and meditation practices. There were some gentle stretching exercises to get our systems going and to build up our muscle groups but we took these very slowly and at our own pace. Sometimes I over-estimated my capability and did too much, but that was usually because I was trying to keep up with someone who had a higher level of ability. The first rule of yoga is to listen to the body and work with it, not against it!

That year I started visiting the Yoga for Health Foundation in Bedfordshire, then the largest residential centre of its kind in Europe. They were doing a lot of work with ME as well as courses for people living with other chronic conditions. Here I also learned more about the importance of proper diet and the value of meditation in quieting the mind.

During my time studying and practising yoga at the Centre, the improvement in my health was so dramatic that I realised yoga was having a profound effect on my wellbeing. Pranayama, or yoga breathing (through the nose from the diaphragm, rather than rapidly and from the upper chest as we tend to do when stressed) was really important in my journey back to health, as were the relaxation and stretching postures I practiced daily. Gradually I became physically stronger. I also became more spiritually aware as the more I practised yoga, the more I was getting in touch with the 'real' Fiona.

In studying yoga philosophy, I've tried to incorporate its moral codes of conduct into my every day life, which include 'non violence' and compassion towards all living beings in thought, word and deed. Like many people with ME I always had an overactive mind that was, no doubt, over-stimulating my nervous system. For this reason, I was also interested to learn the extent to which yoga is about controlling the mind to help you live in the moment.

Staying in the here and now reduces tension and helps me feel much calmer about the future. For example, if I had a relapse, I used to panic about how that would affect me, what I would have to cancel and not be able to do. This worry would then lead to further illness and exhaustion. By learning to surrender – a key lesson in yoga – I was able to just accept that this is how I was for the time being and let go of any anxieties about the future. I could choose to be ill and unhappy, or ill for now, and happy. This state of mind got me out of relapse faster than any pill I could have popped.

By 1999 I was beginning to teach yoga to other people with ME and embarked on a teacher-training course with the Yoga for Health Foundation. Then in 2003 I was contacted by Alex Howard who wanted to interview me for a set of CDs he was making. They were produced to tie into "Why ME?" a book detailing his own slow journey towards recovery. Alex's message, which I had understood intellectually but not actually put into action, was that if you want to get better, then you have to live an authentic and happy life. This really resonated with me. The idea that we should avoid situations and choices that make us more ill, and focus on doing what makes us feel better. At around the same time I read Ekhart Tolle's "The Power of Now", which I continue to refer to and be inspired by.

In 2004 I left my marriage after twenty-four years. The lessons I'd learnt through studying yoga philosophy had woken me up. I'd been locked for years in a destructive relationship with a controlling man who had a drink problem, which left me permanently on edge. I realised I would never achieve the peace of mind and quality of life I wanted as long as I was trapped in an unhappy relationship where I didn't feel able to be myself. However, in making this difficult choice I was leaving behind a comfortable and safe existence – no money worries and a beautiful home in the country. It took all my strength and courage to jump from the known to the unknown. Things were very difficult with the divorce, but the relief at being free was overwhelming, and, not surprisingly, my health improved just from being out of this stressful relationship

With little money and nowhere to live, I had no idea what I would do or how I would survive. I was forty-eight with no real job prospects and my health was, at best, unreliable. Most days were good but I had to pace myself carefully. My brother and his family took me in until I was offered a live-in job at the Yoga for Health Foundation, cooking and doing a bit of teaching. I loved working at the Yoga for Health Centre but still lacked confidence. My ex-husband had spent many years putting me down so I thought I would never have a relationship with anyone again. However, I met another yoga teacher at the Centre and, to my amazement, soon found myself in a relationship with him.

At the beginning of 2005 I went to do some more teaching in India. My health was really good now. The food and sunshine clearly agreed with me, as did the three hours of yoga I was able to do every day. However, the first retreat I worked at was run by a woman who was heavily into drugs, so I plucked up the courage to leave, again not knowing what would become of me. After a week, I found another retreat where I was offered a bit of teaching and also free training in Reiki, a form of healing. To my surprise I met four other people with ME there – it seemed to draw people who wanted to try and recover in the sunshine.

I could hardly believe that this was my new life. From having been trapped in a wheelchair I was now beginning to really live again!

I had to return to England to finalise my divorce, and decided to move to London, although at this point I had no job and didn't know many people there. Again, I was very lucky. My mum lent me money pending the divorce settlement and an English friend I'd made in India offered me a room to rent and some yoga teaching at her holistic centre in West London.

In June 2005 I relapsed quite badly, becoming bed-bound for a short period. I went to my mother's to recover, desperately afraid that everything I was building up was going to collapse. However, by meditating, focusing only on the present moment and refusing to give in to panic, I stabilised again. I then had two court cases to get through plus dealing with selling our house and storing my furniture. Through judicious pacing and taking on just one task at a time, I managed. I was then offered more and more yoga classes so that by the time my divorce came through I was teaching fifteen sessions a week.

Considering I had been in a wheelchair ten years before, I think that what I'm able to sustain these days shows how profound the healing effect of yoga can be. I am fifty now but have my independence and health and am able to cope with a physically demanding job – albeit one I love.

I haven't had a major setback since June 2005 and, providing I am careful, my health is good. Okay, so I don't party every night, but I have an excellent quality of life. I have learned a lot more about prana (a Sanskrit word meaning 'universal energy') since the first edition of my book *Beat Fatigue with Yoga* was published back in 1999. For instance, one could update yoga philosophy on quieting the mind by saying that too much materialism, or overloading of the senses through continual TV, noise or stimulation, wears us down and takes us away from our spiritual core.

People often ask how I've reached an almost full recovery from ME in case they can use anything from my experience. Obviously I practice yoga regularly - especially meditation and slow breathing from the diaphragm. Most people with ME who attend my yoga classes come in breathing too fast from the upper chest, which exacerbates muscle aches, low energy and poor sleep. I also try and live in the present moment, eat healthy whole foods, only make constructive relationships with people who are positive, and not to fritter away energy by overloading the senses with too much shopping, computing, or television.

There's nothing holding me back now. A group of us are currently involved in setting up a new charity to replace the old The Yoga for Health Foundation Centre which was sadly forced to close. I plan to return to India for a few months' backpacking next year and from there, who knows?

Most useful aid to recovery - yoga

Recommended websites
www.theoptimumhealthclinic.com
chronobiologyuk@yahoo.co.uk
www.asquith.ltd.co.uk
www.brainfog.org
www.meassociation.org.uk
www.info@revival.co.uk
www.afme.org.uk

Useful contact - Angela Stevens has excellent cassette tapes and CDs with yoga for M.E. sessions on them. Angela also keeps a list of teachers across the UK who specialise in teaching yoga for M.E. so if you want to know if there is a teacher in your area send an SAE to: Angela Stevens, Laminga, Southview Road, Wadhurst, East Sussex, UK TN5 6TL

Fiona's advice - give yourself time and love and be gentle with your body – pace yourself. Accept what *is* for now. And most of all, try to find your spiritual core, in whatever way works for you.

Fiona Agombar

Christine's Story

You *can* eat yourself well

I was ill for ten years, with my symptoms masked by anti-depressants and sleeping pills. I even spent time in a mental hospital while I was swopped from one anti-depressant to another. I eventually deteriorated hugely with great exhaustion and depression. I decided that I should get off the drugs and started withdrawing from them slowly over a year. I had been diagnosed with M.E.

One day I was directed by friends and a local homeopath to read a book - which in a matter of weeks began a complete turn-around in my health. My cloudy and depressed mind cleared and my exhaustion was replaced by energy.

This book was a book written by the nutritionist Erica White, "Beat Candida Cook Book – Four Point Plan to Beat Candidiasis". Erica White has also written a book called "Beat Fatigue Handbook" specifically for ME sufferers.

I was amazed, as were my family and friends, at the transformation in my health after just a few weeks into the initial stages of the Four Point Plan. From being slumped in a chair exhausted, and with little interest in life, I was writing Christmas cards, putting up decorations and cooking for my husband. This was in December 2003. Staying on the diet the improvement continued, and has been maintained. Now I am leading a full, healthy and happy life again.

Erica White suffered ill health herself for many years and found a cure in a strict change of diet and the taking of supplements. She went on to become a qualified nutritionist with her own clinic in Essex. From 2002 to 2004 with the approval of the Local Research Ethics Committee she ran a research project on Chronic Fatigue Syndrome/ ME, which has been accepted for publication by the internationally renowned Journal of Orthomolecular Medicine and is just about to be published.

Although since May 2006 she has retired from her clinic to devote her time to lecturing in this country and abroad, a web site now continues to offer the services of her programme which will be tailored specifically to meet each individual's needs (see below).

I hope that this information and my experience can be useful to other people. You *can* eat yourself well.

Most useful aid to recovery – anti-candida diet

Recommended books - "Beat Candida Cook Book – Four Point Plan to Beat Candidiasis"
by Erica White. "Beat Fatigue Handbook" by Erica White

Recommended website - www.nutritionhelp.com

Christine Whiteman

Louise's Story

Acknowledge that the body/mind does exist and take notice!

In general my life was ticking along just fine. In fact the past couple of years were more settled than ever before with regard to my health, home, family and working circumstances. All the things that I felt were important were in place. I had been happily married for many years with two children. We had a nice home, my husband had a secure job and I worked part-time to give myself some financial independence and to enable me to splash out on those little luxuries that we all like to have. My physical health had always been good but in the past I had suffered from depression and anxiety. Following treatment I had been given the opportunity of a job working with people I knew, and so I put my efforts into this and it helped me to virtually overcome these problems.

Two years later there was a short period of time when I found I wasn't feeling quite as well as usual, but it didn't affect me enough to focus my attention on it. I worked in a stressful environment and it was our busiest time of year. I found that I wasn't sleeping very well; either I took a long while to go to sleep or I would wake up at around 4 am and not be able to get back to sleep again. This wasn't a nightly occurrence but it would happen a few times each week.

As time progressed I became more tired. I sometimes experienced mild feelings of anxiety for no apparent reason and occasionally I would suddenly have what I can only describe as a 'hot flush'. I was soon to be forty so I honestly thought that maybe I was already on 'the change'!

A few weeks later the school summer holidays commenced. My husband's work takes him away from home for periods of up to six weeks at a time and his rota meant that he would be away for the duration. Usually he is able to spend some of the holiday period at home and so together we take care of the children and we go out as a family.

My husband's support in this way is invaluable to me, particularly because my son, aged nine, has attention deficit disorder. He has short term memory problems and lack of concentration. He often becomes impatient and short tempered when he is unable to focus on tasks that he can't complete and he becomes bored very easily. He can only concentrate on an activity for a short period of time before he needs to change to something different to occupy him, and he's never happy playing by himself.

He's not so hyperactive now, although he is still often very energetic and noisy! However, he has a wonderful vibrant personality, full of humour and one which most people describe as, "having character". He is also a very loving and affectionate little boy.

My daughter was then aged fourteen and she was exhibiting the independent side of her character like most teenagers do! There was nothing particularly serious going on and I have to say that generally she is a very sensible young lady. It's just that there were many disagreements between us. Some of the issues included an untidy bedroom, expecting a taxi service on tap and an unlimited supply of money to facilitate all the outings and activities she wanted to take part in. Sometimes it caused an atmosphere in the house which was neither relaxed nor pleasant. However, this phase didn't go on for too long because we discussed everything and we came to an understanding with regard to the issues concerned.

Those few months were more difficult for me than normal, but they were not as stressful as other times in my life when I've had more serious things to deal with. Even so I was struggling and I couldn't find a solution to ease the situation. I kept my feelings to myself instead of talking about them. My husband was away from home and during school holidays I don't have the normal opportunities to meet with my friends. Therefore, I felt frustrated, alone and somewhat trapped in my situation. There were other people I could have told, but I really thought that I should be able to cope; it was something quite trivial, and so I should just get on with it and not complain. After all, there are many people in far worse situations than mine. I had a lot to be thankful for and happy about, so I had no right to feel this way. I tried to ignore my feelings and carry on regardless. This included ignoring the mild symptoms I was experiencing.

The children went back to school and my husband returned from work. Things should definitely become easier, but suddenly I felt exhausted and ill. My husband and I went into the city to look around the shops but after a couple of hours I desperately needed to sit down. Suddenly I felt extremely tired and weak, so much so that I was unable to continue what we were doing. There was a cafe nearby and so we decided to go there straightaway so that I could sit down and have lunch. I thought maybe having something to eat would be all that was required for me to feel better. However, nothing improved and so we went home.

The next few days I thought I was coming down with a bug or flu because I still felt tired and ill, but nothing more specific than that. Then I became worse. I developed a severe sore throat and felt so ill that I didn't want to get out of bed and I stayed there for the majority of the day and night. I also noticed that I had intermittent joint pain in most of the joints in my body. I didn't see the doctor until about two weeks later when I was diagnosed with tonsillitis. I had never suffered from this before and I thought that within another couple of weeks I would be better and I would be able to return to work. Not so!

When I expected the symptoms to improve, they became worse and I developed even more varying symptoms. When I saw my doctor again I was told that I had a virus. The strangest thing was that the symptoms would fluctuate in severity from hour to hour; I may feel all of them at the same time or only a few of them. The list of symptoms I experienced comprises of fatigue, sore throat, swollen glands, muscle pain, multi joint pain, muscle weakness, high temperature, low temperature, insomnia, hypersomnia, very poor concentration and short term memory loss. The fatigue was there permanently.

At best it was bearable, the way anyone would feel the next day after a very poor night's sleep and at its worst I was completely and utterly exhausted to such a degree that functioning of any sort was impossible. The other symptoms would come and go in varying degrees of severity but I was never free from them all. In particular I was surprised how my throat could be perfectly fine but within a minute it could change and become extremely sore. It would remain sore for a few hours or many days and then all of a sudden it would be fine again.

It was exactly the same with the joint and muscle pain. If I was experiencing a 'good' day I would always try to make the most of it by catching up on housework, or popping out somewhere locally, just to get out of the house for a change. The day may start off pretty well but within hours it could all change. Several times I experienced a sudden wave of total exhaustion. When this happened I couldn't even think what I was doing, let alone do anything physical. It was so severe, that I felt if I didn't get to bed and lie down within ten minutes then I would die.

As for the poor concentration levels I became very frustrated. I was unable to read for more than a quarter of an hour without experiencing exhaustion and even holding a conversation could be difficult. My brain would become a complete blur, I wouldn't be able to follow what I was reading/listening to/talking about, and my thinking would become very muddled.

The short term memory loss I experienced was frightening. I found myself doing such stupid things around the house so that sometimes I thought I was losing my mind altogether! Some examples are putting dishwasher tablets in the washing machine, and loading up the dishwasher with dirty utensils when I hadn't finished removing all the clean ones first. One day I was looking all around the house for my cup of tea, which I knew I had made only a couple of minutes ago, only to realise that I only got as far as boiling the kettle.

Another time I had something important to send abroad. I weighed it and put all the necessary labels on and went to the post box just around the corner from my house. As soon as I returned home I realised I had missed something vitally important; I hadn't put the stamps on! AARRGG! It was a few minutes before the post box was due to be emptied, but I couldn't exert myself anymore to go back there, so my husband went instead, rescued the package and put the postage on! Fortunately I never did anything that had serious consequences. I know we can all be absent minded sometimes, but it's a worry when it's a daily occurrence and you wonder what totally stupid thing you are going to do next. You are living in a "fog," which is why it is often referred to as brain fog. You're going through the motions but you don't have a clue what you are doing, or otherwise you think you know what you're doing but realise sooner or later that you're doing it all wrong.

My diminished temperature control meant that I suffered from high temperatures sometimes, but mostly I felt very cold all the time. My family would be surprised to see me huddled on the settee in a sleeping bag, the fire on full as well as having the heating on! For me, it was the only way I could feel comfortably warm.

After a few weeks of becoming ill, my doctor told me that it sounded like I had post viral fatigue. Blood tests were done to check for anything else, but they all came back negative. During this period of time, when I was able to sit at the computer, I was searching the medical websites on the internet, trying to glean more information and work out what illness I had. All sorts of possibilities became apparent. Many of my symptoms could be attributed to a variety of illnesses, including lupus, multiple sclerosis, and leukaemia. It was a very worrying time, knowing you feel so ill, but not having a diagnosis, though I concluded that the most likely illness I had was ME. Within three months my doctor referred me to an ME clinic and told me I would wait a minimum of approximately six months to see a specialist there. By then I had read quite a lot of material on the internet about the illness and it all looked very bleak indeed. I didn't have what most people would class as a 'serious' illness or something terminal but it seemed that there was no cure and most people had the illness for many years, so as far as I was concerned this was serious! It seemed the best news was that you don't die from it. Well, I thought, "YIPPEE!" However, I since learned that it's not strictly true because some people find the pain and suffering so unbearable that they commit suicide.

There are also emotional issues to deal with, which are unexpected and often very frustrating and upsetting to experience. The cause is lack of understanding by other people regarding ME and how it affects sufferers. Surprisingly, even many doctors don't accept that the illness exists, though I didn't experience this. Fortunately for me, my doctor, my family and friends were understanding and supportive and I am very appreciative of this.

Some peoples' thoughts are, "Isn't it time you were back at work?" Certainly if I had felt well enough to be at work then I would have returned straight away. I have never been a skiver and in two years of working in my job I had only had about three days off sick in total. Had I simply not wanted to work, I could have resigned, because I wasn't reliant on the income from it. I only worked two days each week and it was for my own personal satisfaction. Other comments: "Oh, yeah, I feel tired all the time; I know what it's like!" "Isn't it that yuppie flu thing?" "Well, at least some people do recover from it, don't they? So that's good news." All these comments trivialise the severity of the symptoms. People seem to have no idea of the extreme exhaustion experienced, even the medical term, "fatigue" is a huge understatement. It's not simply "feeling tired all the time," which is the misconception that most people have. It's a level of exhaustion which can prevent you from functioning physically and mentally.

One day my husband and I went out, but within an hour I became very tired and we had to make our way back home. In the car we were having a general conversation. I knew my head felt all fuzzy and I didn't seem able to take in all that he was saying. Then he told me that I was talking complete gobble-de-gook and asked me if I realised. Yes, I did! I was having difficulty listening, comprehending and responding. Even when I was speaking my words were coming out all muddled up. I don't think that anyone can fully realise what it's like unless they have the illness themselves.

I know this will sound cruel, but I sometimes wished that people would experience the illness at its worst and its affects just for one day in their life. Then they would be able to understand what it's like to live with and could imagine the impact of feeling that way for many months or years.

The best advice I had was to rest as much as I needed to, never overdo things, certainly try not to become stressed and to try relaxation techniques. I bought some CDs with relaxation music and meditations and they did help with relaxation.

I read about alternative treatments in the hope of finding something to help me feel better. I had already started eating more healthy meals but I also decided to change to a yeast free, low sugar diet. I took various vitamins and supplements, but I didn't experience any relief in my symptoms at all.

I bought a gym ball and stretch band which came in a package with a video tape demonstrating very gentle Pilates movements. It was good to have something at home that I could do in my own time whenever I felt able to, even if I only managed five minutes. I hoped it would help to prevent any long term muscle weakness.

A few months later I found out about Reiki. For me it provided the deepest form of relaxation I had ever experienced. After a couple of sessions I noticed some improvement in my energy levels, memory and concentration.

By then I had been away from work for five months and even though it was justified, I felt guilty about being off sick for so long. Therefore, I decided now was the time to go back, even though I had only experienced an improved spell for about three weeks. I arranged with my manager to start back on half my hours. It wasn't too busy at this time of year and so there wasn't so much pressure. I only had to work two mornings a week, from 9am to 1 pm, and with the days being Tuesday and Friday, I had ample time to rest in between. Surely this wasn't going to be too much of a problem?

During the first month I muddled through, but as soon as I came home I was totally exhausted and would go straight to bed. I would continue to rest as much as possible during my days off and I was having difficulty keeping on top of normal household tasks. Usually I slept all afternoon in order to get through the day. Muscle and joint pain became more severe and my GP increased the dosage of amitriptyline to try and alleviate the muscle pain. However, as soon as I took 30 mg the sedative effect was too high and I felt like a zombie day and night. I decided to decrease the dosage and put up with the pain rather than increase medication even more.

Before long I felt under pressure to increase my working hours. Other people didn't realise how difficult it was for me. I can't say I blame them because I didn't look ill and I'm not a person who moans about how I feel. I didn't tell my friends how ill I felt and whenever I saw them, which wasn't very often, it had to be arranged at the last minute, according to what kind of day I was having and therefore they never saw me at my worst.

Anyway, I decided that my job was so important to me that I would work my two full days a week as contracted. I was very stubborn and I didn't want this illness to get the better of me. I don't really know why but I convinced myself that I just had to soldier on and eventually I would get better. I kept thinking, "Just get through this week and then I may turn the corner, this can't last forever."

Before I became ill my husband and I had booked a special holiday. For the first time we were able to make arrangements for the children to be looked after, so it was just the two of us. As the holiday approached I was worried that I would be too ill to go. My family thought that I should postpone it "until you're better." I had a dilemma deciding what to do. I knew I was too ill to enjoy the holiday properly but I honestly thought that the illness may get worse and so this could be my last chance to go. I took the stubborn approach again and I was determined that we would go, even if we had to compromise on our plans. As the holiday approached I took a week off prior to going away in order to gain plenty of rest and to give me the best chance of being well enough to go.

To my surprise it all went better than expected. The symptoms were definitely less severe, though still present and toward the end of the holiday the fatigue, muscle pain and joint pain decreased. My symptoms didn't become as severe as I thought they would and so I decided that from now on I would ignore them and carry on doing all the things that I wanted to do. With renewed positive thinking I returned to work. On my first day back the pain I was experiencing started to increase. I tried to ignore it and carry on. This went on for a couple of weeks, during which time the symptoms were increasing by the day.

I continued looking for alternative treatments because I was becoming depressed and frightened that the illness would become even worse and that I would soon be confined to bed. However, the number of so called 'cures' out there, all costing various amounts of money, is unbelievable. At one time I didn't know which way to turn and I simply 'froze' and did nothing for a while, feeling ever more confused and despondent.

A month before I went on holiday I heard about a treatment called Mickel Therapy. Fortunately there was a Mickel Therapist nearby. After my very first appointment I felt far more positive than I had in a very long time. Almost immediately I was able to address an issue that was affecting me and the severity of my symptoms started to decrease within a few days. I kept a journal which enabled me and the therapist to understand what the 'symptom message' was. From then on as I applied the principles, the symptoms continued decreasing and what amazed me most is that it wasn't long before the severe joint and muscle pain I had been experiencing ceased completely. For me this was incredible!

In keeping the journal I realised that my symptoms became worse when I was at work or a few hours prior to going into work. The stressful environment was having a greater affect than I could ever have imagined! It became crystal clear to me that the stressful environment was too much and for the first time I admitted to myself that even though I liked my job, I had to leave. Without Mickel Therapy I am certain that I wouldn't have recognised my job as being a major contributory factor with regard to my illness.

This was my turning point. The hypothalamitis theory taught me that my symptoms were there to remind me not to ignore my feelings anymore, but to acknowledge them and address them accordingly. The other issues I had to address were related to home life. I certainly needed to ensure I had time for myself again. There were a couple of other issues related to home life that I needed to take action on, and as I did so, symptoms just continued decreasing until soon they *all* ceased!

I made arrangements so I could take a break from dealing with the children and to relieve pressure by handling things in a more positive and beneficial way.

I found childcare for my son so that during school holidays I could have a day off each week to do whatever I wanted, whether it was to relax at home or go out with friends. It also benefited him because he had other children to play with and plenty to occupy him and so he was very happy with the arrangement. My husband changed his job and was home every weekend, which was a great improvement for us all. He was becoming more unhappy about spending long periods away, so it was a good move for himself as well as the family. The more I took notice of my true feelings, acknowledged the issues I wasn't happy about and then made positive changes, the more the symptoms decreased and the better I felt, and as time progressed the symptoms ceased altogether. This was achieved with four sessions of therapy, over a period of two months, and then one last follow up appointment.

Since then I've had no return of my symptoms at all! I have been leading a normal busy life, taking care of the home and family and I've also started working again, but for a different company, in a job which has better conditions and environment.

I am aware that I need to continue applying the principles of the therapy in order to prevent symptoms returning. Now I take notice of my true feelings instead of ignoring them. If I'm uncomfortable or stressed about something in particular then I actively seek a solution which will relieve the pressure. Of course some situations are more easily dealt with than others. However, a key point is to recognise what your body is telling you and acknowledge this instead of burying your head in the sand and continuing regardless; when you do that you're setting yourself up for problems.

I now eat a healthier diet than I did prior to the illness. Also, I make time for myself, which I use for enjoyment and relaxation. Sometimes this involves setting an hour aside to listen to relaxation music, meditation or self-treating with Reiki. Periodically, I also see my Reiki Master for a session of pure relaxation, particularly if I feel stressed. I'm in perfect health and I see no reason why it shouldn't continue.

It's great to get my life back on track, be as active as I want to be, able to make plans and to feel positive about the future. I can enjoy going on holiday again, distance is no problem, the travelling not having to be restricted. I can participate fully in family life, enjoy days out, and can even spend a whole day shopping with my teenage daughter again! I have a busy weekly routine going to work and keeping up with all the household chores, but I still find time to socialise with friends. It's great to be able to do all of this, to feel happy, and not to be struggling through life anymore.

Most useful aid to recovery - Mickel Therapy

Recommended websites
www.mickeltherapy.com
www.sleepydust.net

Louise's advice - for everyone reading this, I'd like to impress on you not to give up hope.

Louise

Monique's Story

Pay it forward

Before my ME I was super fit, full of energy, athletic and always on the go. People use to say "no flies would ever land on Monique!" and this was true.

However things changed.

When I first had ME it started with, what I thought, was a bad case of flu. It was 1993, I was thirty years old and I was living in the U.K. I was under a lot of stress at the time because my father had had a severe accident, and the consequences meant that my family lost their business and home and I had to find alternative work. During that bout of 'flu' I stayed at home for only two days, although I felt really awful, because in Britain one can't spend many days off sick - you could be sacked for it. From that time onwards my health went downhill and a visit to a homeopath in Wales confirmed that I had ME. I had to continue working even though I was ill, and I could never let on to my colleagues that I was unwell, as I simply couldn't afford to lose my job.

After years of working the typical British sixty to seventy hour week, my husband and I decided to move back to Holland. I visited homeopathic doctors in Holland and Germany but they couldn't help. The homeopath in Germany tested my blood and said that I had an abnormal amount of white blood cells in my blood. Obviously my exhausted body was still trying to fight a virus.

My beloved father died in January 2002 and my ME became progressively worse. It is a known fact that emotions can really have a bad effect on ME. I was really in a terrible state by July 2004. My ME had never been so bad. It was the first time I was really scared as the ME had affected my legs and I could hardly walk. All my organs inside were churning and I lay on my bed desperately wondering what I could do. I was frightened. I was scared I would end up in a wheelchair.

In the early stages when I first had ME.my arms were like lead and to try and cycle was almost impossible. I was always sweating with the least exertion during all sorts of weather and this continued for eleven years. I felt I was getting weaker with every year. I tried all I could to help myself fight it, but at the end of the day, as a layman, I didn't have the medical knowledge to know what to do or how to help myself.

One day a good friend of mine gave me a book, "Heden ik" written by a Dutch writer called Renate Dorrestein. This book explained how Renate had had ME and had tried all sorts of doctors and quacks in desperation to get better, before discovering an orthomolecular doctor, which resulted in her consequent recovery. I couldn't put the book down. I had never heard of such a doctor before! However, there are many more orthomolecular doctors here in Holland than in the U.K. Orthomolecular doctors prevent and treat disease by correcting imbalances and deficiencies in the body of vitamins, minerals, amino acids and essential fatty acids - and people with ME are often found to have problems in these areas.

Fortunately for me there was an orthomolecular doctor who worked in a neighbouring village near to where I lived. I visited her for the first time in July 2004. She gave me a thorough physical examination and I had urine and faecal tests. She also did numerous thorough blood tests. She put me on a strict diet of no dairy products, no gluten, no pork and no sugar and introduced me to the Blood Group diet, which I still like to keep to now. She also gave me various supplements like

Vitamin B12 injections, selenium, L-carnitine, essential fatty acids and homeopathic drops.

The doctor really took the time to listen to me, and once I had described my symptoms she told me that she thought I still fighting a virus. I was most impressed, she was not at all like your average family practitioner.

When she got the blood tests back she could see that I did have a virus in my blood and that virus was glandular fever (ziekte van Pffeifer). I had thought it was only a virulent strain of the flu. She gave me homeopathic granules to take over several weeks, in increasingly higher potencies. It brought all the symptoms back at first, but eventually I noticed that the constant low-grade fever had gone.

Having instigated the changes in my diet I felt generally better. ME as many fellow patients will know, had affected all my internal organs - liver, kidneys, pancreas, adrenal glands and so on. My thyroid was not working well and she had given me tablets to help that problem too.

We moved house on 1st November 2004. I told her I was concerned that I would not have the energy for that. She recommended that I take a relatively new product Artenox D (three times daily with each meal) and Artenox M (one daily in the morning with breakfast). These tablets were like rocket fuel. What an energy boost!

After visiting the doctor every two months for a year, in April 2005 she confirmed what I already knew - I was cured!

Although eleven years older my energy levels are now what they used to be before I was ill. I really feel I have been given a second chance in life! I am so grateful that Renate did something positive about her ME by writing about her experiences in a book which led to my recovery. A friend of mine told my story to a recently widowed friend who also has ME. Her friend is now going to visit my orthomolecular doctor. I hope that maybe I can contribute something positive from my experience - like the film "Pay it Forward".

It is just wonderful to have my energy back again! I am now busy with my final exams for Interior Design and I am presently talking to a local contractor about working with them. Currently we are having our home renovated. I can paint and decorate again and participate in everything. My design work on our home will be a good advertisement for me. I have also had the energy to help my mother who has been ill. I could never have helped her if I still had ME.

It is so fantastic to be able to move swiftly, work physically hard, enjoy dancing, gardening, think clearly and travel with no more exhaustion. Now I have my life back again. My husband no longer has to do the shopping and cleaning. It is so great to be fit - what price can you put on your health? I wish to thank my darling husband for his loving devotion and support during my illness.

Most useful aid to recovery - Orthomolecular medicine

Recommended book - "Heden ik" by Renate Doreestein IBSN: 9025402267

Recommended websites
www.orthomolecular.org
www.ortho.nl.

Monique's advice - always question everything and never, ever give up!

Monique

Helen's Story

The biggest breakthrough was a wheat and dairy-free diet

At her worst my daughter, Helen, got to as low as 20%. I know every case is different, every patient has slightly different symptoms, and that what helps one individual may not help another; but I decided it was worth writing our story in case others could benefit from our experiences and/or gain hope for recovery themselves.

We moved to Tonbridge from London six years ago mainly because we were keen to live in a clean environment with less traffic. Before we left London Helen had a constant slight sniffle but was otherwise healthy.

Our new house was fumigated for fleas shortly after we moved in and the car park next door was sprayed with some kind of pesticide.

We didn'ot immediately settle in Tonbridge. Both children found the new primary school boring and old-fashioned and Peter really hated it. Helen was quieter about her dislike of the school but made a couple of friends.

After one year she went to secondary school. She appeared to cope exceptionally well and worked hard. She liked the school. She was rather serious at this time but otherwise well, apart from increasing sniffles - for which the GP prescribed a nasal spray. Towards the end of the first year there she developed an illness involving swollen glands and tiredness. Blood tests did not show glandular fever. There was no treatment. Around this time we consulted a lay homeopath, Marta, who prescribed remedies which did help the sniffles and catarrh.

The following year Helen began to get severe stomach pains after every meal. She was also very tired. The GP referred us to a pediatrician who diagnosed constipation. This was a surprise, as Helen's diet had always included lots of fruit and vegetables, beans, and fluids. Also, although not sporty, she had exercise walking to and from school. Laxatives and antacids helped slightly but the problem persisted. Helen started to attend school for only half days and had to rest in the afternoons. She was too tired for any social life or fun.

We went back to the pediatrician who diagnosed CFS. There was a brief ten minute explanation of the illness and we were told she would improve gradually over the next 18 eighteen months. We found the diagnosis of CFS confusing and were unsure whether this was the same thing as ME or not. Eventually we decided it was. A friend put me in touch with Action for ME. At first I read their magazines quietly and kept them away from Helen, as I think I was in some sort of denial,and was worried that she would find pictures of people more severely affected upsetting. I was still clinging to the hope that she was only mildly affected and would recover within 18 months, as the pediatrician had said.

Helen tried to improve gradually - but only became more and more tired. The stomach pains after eating continued and she had frequent colds. I told our GP that the only thing that had seemed to help was homeopathy, and she referred her to an NHS homeopathic doctor in Tunbridge Wells instead of the lay homeopath. Helen became more and more unwell over the next few months, until finally she caught a bad cold, which she never really got over. We went back to the pediatrician, who said she would have to do even less. Helen was too ill to go to school at all and became very depressed. She spent the next couple of days crying.

It was at this time that we decided to try anything and everything as NHS conventional treatment had let us down. We tried anything that was not dangerous and did not make Helen even more worn out from traveling.

I asked the lay homeopath, Marta, to see Helen again, instead of traveling to the doctor's homeopath in Tunbridge Wells. She was wonderful and agreed to see Helen at home. She prescribed a different set of remedies and promised to keep in touch by email as she was going abroad.

A friend suggested kinesiology to check for food allergies. The kinesiologist said that Helen was allergic to brazil nuts and lettuce (one of the most heavily sprayed crops). She prescribed some expensive vitamin and mineral supplements.

Another friend suggested reflexology. We found a reflexologist, Alyson, in the next street, and Helen had treatment there weekly, then fortnightly, then monthly, until about nine months ago. She pinpointed the main tender area to be around the hypothalamus in the brain and also found thyroid and gut areas to be tender. I shared this information with Marta and our GP. Marta prescribed remedies including hypothalamus, pituitary and pineal gland in potency, as problems in this area also seemed strongly linked with clinical signs - tiredness, coldness and poor immunity. We also started on an organic diet.

I feel sure that both the reflexology and these homeopathic remedies helped. After each treatment Helen would drink a lot of water and then sleep. She would often start shivering and get flushed after the first treatments. Marta explained that this could be the body trying to reset its temperature control.

Alyson, the reflexologist, taught me to massage Helen's stomach with oil below the umbilicus in a clockwise direction for 10 minutes each night. This worked better for relieving the constipation than any laxatives!

For about a year Helen was unable to leave the house except to sit in the garden. She could travel to the reflexologist by car, as I could park right outside the door. Visiting the GP or the hospital was almost impossible, as it is quite a walk from the car park to the consulting room. Our GP thought a wheelchair was a bad idea but did support my application for a blue disabled parking badge. On occasions I guiltily borrowed a wheelchair from the Red Cross, such as when we went to the hospital outpatient department. Helen did not like sitting in a wheelchair.

For our summer holiday we hired a boat on the river. This enabled her to sit and watch the world go by without moving far from her bed and look normal to passing boaters. We didn't go shopping. Helen chose clothes from a home shopping catalogue. Her only pleasures at this time were stroking her rabbits, lying in the sun, and listening to music -played very quietly as noise hurt her ears. The council eventually provided a home tutor, but this was more of a social than an educational occasion as Helen was really too ill to learn.

We had read about the importance of graded exercise and knew it was important not to let the joints stiffen up so another thing we tried was yoga. We bought some audio tapes especially for people with ME from a yoga teacher called Angela Stevens. These were very gentle exercises that you can do in bed at a slow pace. They also included visualization exercises that helped you to imagine yourself away, outside of your situation. Each day we tried to walk a few steps along the street before sitting down on the garden wall - but this was hard for Helen and progress was painfully slow.

Someone else put us in touch with Action for ME and AYME (Action for young people with ME). Now Helen also looked at their magazines. I was worried that they would drag her down further but she said it was a help for her to know that there were other children in her position. At this time, she says that she worried that she was going mad. I felt guilty and worried that poor parenting on my part had made her psychologically ill. One of my sisters was diagnosed with CFS/ME soon after Helen and this intensified the idea that the problem was mine and from my side of the family.

I was working fewer hours than my husband and so was more often at home. I had the role of main carer and took her to the various health care appointments. My husband became more and more distant during

Helen's illness and seemed to blame her for being ill. Whenever I went out to work and he was the carer I would come home and listen to each complain about the other. He complained that she did not say 'thank you' when he did things for her. She complained that he was too noisy and rushed her. I was stuck in the middle with a headache.

I asked our GP to refer us to family therapy and told my husband that it was because I was fed up and could not cope this way any longer. The three of us attended two joint sessions at the hospital with a psychiatrist and a psychologist. Her brother was in school. We brought Helen from the car park in a wheelchair, borrowed from the red cross, and asked if she could lie down through the session. The third session was cancelled as one of the doctors was ill. Helen was very pleased not to have to travel there and my husband suggested that we should not go again as it was obviously so upsetting and tiring for Helen. I agreed to this as things seemed to have settled down between them at home.

The breakthrough came when we discovered Helen's food intolerances. Helen wanted to try a wheat and dairy free diet, as she had heard it sometimes helped ME. At first I was not too keen but I agreed to a month's trial. There seemed to be some improvement! Then someone told me about the York Test postal service which does blood checks for food intolerances. This showed up intolerances to gluten, dairy and brazil nuts. The kinesiologist months before had only discovered brazil nuts of these three.

Helen has been on a gluten and dairy free, mainly organic diet ever since then. Her stomach is no longer painful after eating. She has gone from a size six to a size ten and she no longer takes any treatment or medication.

The people at York Test suggest that you may outgrow a food intolerance and after several months be able to gradually reintroduce the offending foods. Helen has had no wish to try this. She is just so happy to feel well that she is not going to risk a relapse.

She gradually started walking further and further each day. She is now taking A'levels at college with a view to going on to university, and works fifteen hours a week at an after-school children's club. She dances to loud music, enjoys a social life and has become a Performance Poet. She has performed at several gigs and open mikes and has her own website*. She has a very full social life and enjoys life to the full.

As I said at the beginning of this article; all cases are different and what worked for us may not work for another ME sufferer. However, if you would like to discuss anything mentioned in this article, please feel free to email me.

Most useful aid to recovery - wheat and dairy-free diet

Recommended websites
www.yorktest.com
www.angela-stevens.co.uk
www.geocities.com/prude_fledgling

Frances Long (Helen's mother)

Paul's Story

I recently ran The Great South Run

I have always been a fairly active person. Certainly from my teens onwards I was extremely sporty with an enthusiastic interest in athletics, or more specifically, running. All through my teens I trained heavily, often over-training, with seemingly endless energy supplies!

At the age of twenty I had my first experience of a debilitating illness when I contracted a particularly vicious strain of glandular fever. It halted all activity and in the following months and years I had several lesser relapses of the virus, which curtailed any further extreme training and hindered my working life too.

In 1994 I achieved a lifelong ambition and opened my own retail clothing business. This was very hard work and meant long tiring hours, par for the course being self-employed, but I was more than happy that I was healthy enough to achieve such demands. However, despite a promising first two years, things didn't work out the way I wanted and the business began to crumble from under me, through no fault of my own. I wasn't in a position to walk away, so I had to endure three years of immense mental pressure and financial meltdown. During this time I was often ill with colds, diarrhoea and many other stress induced symptoms. Finally in January 2000 I was forced to close the shop and I took a mundane job to pay the mounting bills. For about six months I was fine, feeling depressed about what had happened, but physically fine.

Early in summer 2000 I began to feel ill and things quickly took a hold of me; severe fatigue, loss of balance, shivers, swollen glands, panic attacks, severe depression and so on, which at first I thought was a glandular fever relapse. To a degree it was, but the symptoms got more bizarre and more intense, gradually worsening over the course of a year, until I was forced to go sick from work. Several visits to the doctor proved inconclusive and my desperation grew. I had become a complete mess and felt broken physically and mentally.

Rather than wait the six months to see an NHS specialist, I decided to see a private specialist, Dr Goggin, who immediately confirmed what I had worked out for myself, that I had ME. He prescribed Paroxitine, an anti-depressant which specifically dealt with the panic attacks and the anxieties he felt were compounding and helping to fuel this horrendous illness. The first week on the tablets were terrible and got so bad that I phoned the doctor at the hospital to tell him I felt ten times worse. He said he suspected this may happen but that I was to continue taking them. After three weeks I returned to see him and by then I was beginning to show some signs of improvement. At this visit he suggested I begin a plan of graduated exercise. At first I thought he was mad, some days I could barely stand, so, " how can I take exercise?" I thought! However, he convinced me that this was the way forward and that he didn't expect to see me again as I was now on the road to recovery. I was shocked by this, but he made me feel confident and believe in myself. I left his office feeling confident I was finally going to get better and determined to follow his advice.

By this time I had been encouraged by my parents to come and stay with them at their bungalow rather than cooped up in my dingy flat - and how right they were. The better surroundings and being able to sit outside in their garden seemed to help my condition and it was from there that I began a daily walking schedule. On day one I could only walk slowly for about 300 metres, but slowly and surely each day I went further and further. The illness backed off and my confidence and fitness improved, and after three weeks I could walk for about an hour!

It was a combination of the tablets, the stay at my parents and the exercise that somehow things fell into place for the better. I was able to return to work, move back home and begin living a relatively normal life again. Things had improved, but I still had the illness and still got bad days and had to make a firm adjustment to my life. I had to be realistic about what I could and couldn't do and take life slower and pace myself.

That was six years ago and I have been well ever since. I now have a wonderful partner, Kate, who has taken time to read about ME and understand it. I no longer have a dingy flat but Kate and I own a lovely house, and believe it or not I also have my own business again – as a market/street trader - which is a fairly physical job, but this time it's working well! As far as exercise goes, I'm able to run again. I recently ran The Great South Run, which I feel is an amazing comeback!

I don't take my recovery for granted, I eat fairly healthily, drink plenty of water and keep myself fit.

Most useful aid to recovery - acceptance

Paul's advice - I would advise people in the midst of M.E. to 'give in to it, but don't give up'. Keep positive, do what you can do and don't worry too much about what you can't do. Remember, recovery is possible.

Paul

Maggie's Story

Getting well is like putting the
pieces of a jigsaw together

In 1996 I was working part time as a Health Visitor. I had a great life with a wonderful partner and we had two sons aged six and nine. Life was busy, interesting and enjoyable. I was involved in running parenting groups at work, which I really enjoyed, and was a Union rep. We had a fairly active social life and went for long hill walks at weekends. Holidays involved camping or visiting friends and relatives in Scotland, Holland or Germany. My hobby was yoga and I had also taken up regular meditation practice.

Over the course of the previous year or so I had begun to feel terribly ill, although I was not at all fatigued. In particular I suffered repeated bouts of what seemed to be a severe stomach bug, which caused me to have several weeks off work each time. On one occasion I was in such acute pain that I thought I had appendicitis and called the doctor, who as usual reassured me that nothing was wrong. Much later I recognised that this had been a flare up of mesenteric lymphadenopathy. All the lymph nodes in my abdomen, as well as the rest of my body, were sore and swollen for a long time, perhaps years.

I had a continual low grade fever. I had constant diarrhoea and my hair started to fall out. I would wake up most nights with severe pain in my upper abdomen on both sides, which felt as though someone was standing on my stomach. I went to the doctor a number of times, each time leaving with the doctor noting 'patient reassured' on my records. I now feel as though the doctor and I were colluding in denial that I was really ill. Eventually I had to face the facts and I asked for a referral to the hospital for investigations and I was referred to the Infectious Diseases Department.

There followed several investigations at hospital including a string test for Giardia, an intestinal parasite. I knew that I had suffered the symptoms of giardiasis many years before, after a holiday in Romania when I had drunk some very dodgy water, and it seemed to me that I was experiencing many of the same symptoms again. By this point the diarrhoea was the colour of bright green grass!

My consultant agreed that the symptoms suggested giardiasis and even though the string test was negative he agreed to prescribe Metronidazole. The result was fantastic. My low grade fevers stopped, the diarrhoea cleared up and although I was very weak, my energy began to return. I thought I just needed a period of recuperation and then I would be back to normal.

Eventually I thought I was well enough to try a phased return to work, and I remember feeling such joy driving there, thinking I was about to get my life back. However I managed only a couple of weeks before the severe symptoms were back. My doctor gave me a repeat prescription of Metronidazole, but this time my health took a total nose dive.

I began to get neurological symptoms. My right leg would not obey orders and began to drag when I walked. At times my right arm was also affected. Over the next few weeks I became desperately ill and needed to be in bed most of the time. I was absolutely baffled as to what might be wrong with me. All I knew was that I felt absolutely terrible. I had numerous investigations but nothing came up except a very abnormal liver function test after the second course of antibiotics. The consultant couldn't explain what this meant but he did diagnose me with chronic fatigue syndrome. There was nothing he could offer and it was time for me to go away and stop troubling the NHS.

My symptoms went from head to toe, literally. I had a constant severe headache, my eyes were red and gritty and my ears sore and painful. I had photophobia and was acutely sensitive to noise. I had brain fog. I couldn't read more than a few words at a time before forgetting what I'd just read, and anyway my eyes had trouble focusing. I had a sore throat and post-nasal drip all the time. My mouth was full of sores and my tongue was covered in a thick white coating and appeared 'frilly' along the edges. My gums were sore and bled easily and there were black spots on them (symptoms I later learned, of pseudo scurvy). The glands in my neck, armpits and groins were swollen and sore. I felt discomfort around my heart and frequently noticed irregular heartbeats, especially missed beats. My guts were in a terrible state, with pain and frequent diarrhoea and I felt as if I was just not digesting food properly. My abdomen was bloated to the size of an eight month pregnancy and I had a lot of wind. My muscles and joints hurt constantly. I was so weak that at times I had to crawl along on my elbows to get to the bathroom. Sitting in a chair was a huge effort.

I had a few episodes of severe trembling, which came on suddenly and uncontrollably. I was utterly exhausted, but found it really hard to sleep, and when I did finally sleep I would often wake up in a panic from terrible dreams with violent imagery. I was unable to tolerate certain chemicals like traffic fumes. At times I was so ill I really thought I might die.

One day my mother bought a book for me called "Recovering from ME" by Dr. William Collinge. This book was really supportive at a time when I badly needed guidance on what to do next. I realized that I would need to work hard to get myself well and that it might take a long time, but that there was no other option. I vowed inwardly to do everything in my power to get well.

I was very upset about losing my job as work had always been very important to me, but I decided that "my job now was to get better". This thought was a great help in keeping me focused on looking after myself and enabled me to feel that I was doing something positive by lying passively in bed, as this was what I needed to do – not that I had any choice! The support I had from my partner and the rest of my family was crucial to getting me through this very worst phase. My partner took on all the household tasks we had previously shared and made a great effort to keep life as normal as possible for the boys. My Mum was an enormous help and for two years she came twice a week and did all the cleaning for us - probably a lot more than I used to do. I often used to reflect on the fact that in her seventies my Mum was vastly more energetic and strong than I was at that time, despite the thirty years plus age difference.

I found missing social occasions really upsetting but there was not a lot of option. I encouraged my partner to bring back news and titbits of conversations when he was out with friends so I could imagine having been there; in other words, I trained him to gossip! My sister was also a great friend to me during this time. She acted as a bridge between the outside world and me. Having my two sons around gave a really good reason to keep life as normal as possible and provided me with a clear sense of what mattered most to me and why I mattered. Perhaps most importantly all these people who were closest to me never stopped believing in me and helped me to feel that I was valued, even though I felt as though I was of no use to anyone.

I knew from the outset that diet and nutrition would be important in getting well.

I tried to eat a healthy diet with plenty of fresh, lightly cooked vegetables and cut out refined carbohydrates and all refined sugars. I ate a small amount of fruit and drank copious amounts of water.

A turning point occurred early in 1998 when I heard about, and went to see, Dr. Sarah Myhill, who is an expert in the management of ME. One of the things Dr. Myhill said to me early on really stuck in my mind. She said that "getting well was like completing a jigsaw - you had to get all the pieces in the right place at the same time".

On Dr. Myhill's recommendation, and after the appropriate tests, I began the following treatments over the next few months ... herbal treatment for gut parasites, anti-fungal medication, injections of Vitamin B12 and magnesium injections, as my red cell magnesium was found to be low. The effect of the magnesium was dramatic. After the first injection I was able to stand up normally for the first time in nine months and the muscle weakness never became so bad again. Nutritional supplements recommended by Dr. Myhill included a good quality multivitamin/mineral, essential fatty acids and vitamin C and she endorsed my approach to diet, which avoided processed foods, refined carbohydrates and sugars but included plenty of fresh vegetables and sources of high quality protein such as meat and fish, organic when possible.

Thyroid tests showed a borderline low thyroid and so Dr. Myhill prescribed thyroxine which led to an almost immediate all round improvement in symptoms, especially a reduction in brain fog and muscle pain and improved quality of sleep.

I didn't take up Dr. Myhill's suggestion of trying an exclusion diet and it was to be years before I finally discovered that I was intolerant to wheat and eggs. I now think I might have recovered earlier had I cut these foods out sooner. It wasn't until my son developed ME and had a test that showed he had a gluten intolerance that I cut out wheat and noticed an immediate improvement, especially in concentration and energy levels.

I found a book by Gill Jacobs "Treating Candida though Diet" and as a result of reading this book and others, I followed a strict anti-candida diet for about two years, took probiotics of various types and continued to develop my awareness of the importance of nutrition.

Having been a nurse, I was well aware of the principles of rehabilitation and the need to avoid deconditioning through inactivity. I was shocked to have suddenly become so very weak and ill despite my best efforts to look after myself and keep going.

For a long period I simply had no option but to spend a great deal of time lying down in bed. My muscles were so weak it was impossible for me to sit upright without support. To travel in the car I had to be propped up with pillows. Using muscles, such as raising my arm to comb my hair or to hold the telephone, immediately led to pain and loss of function. At times my arms and legs would not seem to get the messages from my brain. I remember looking at my legs, saying "in a minute you WILL move" but the ability to move had become a task requiring massive concentration and willpower, instead of something that happened automatically. With the help of the treatment from Dr. Myhill I was able to increase my activity level. I began to use a re-bounder (mini trampoline) for very short periods.

I would get dressed each day and I developed a set of clothes which were suitable for lying in bed but would appear respectable enough if I had to open the door to the postman. With frequent rests I was able to save up the energy I needed to achieve small tasks spread throughout the day. I learned what I could do without causing a set back. Exceeding my limit would lead to days of feeling even worse with flu-like symptoms and aching muscles, so my body trained me in what is now called "pacing". When I became able I began to take a short walk most days, on the level outside the house. I began to do small household tasks such as simple cooking. That way I felt I was being useful to my family and it gave me an achievable goal each day.

During the year preceding my illness, I had lost a large filling that I had partially swallowed. I had had this replaced with another mercury amalgam filling. It was immediately after this that my health sharply declined. I had not noticed the connection at the time but when I began to read about mercury being a possible contributor to chronic health problems I decided to find a dentist who would safely remove and replace my amalgam fillings with a safer compound. I had this done over a two year period, two fillings at a time every six months. It is impossible to know whether this helped me to recover or not, but I am glad I had it done, because it might have helped.

As I slowly improved I found that the delay between overdoing it and the payback grew longer, up to three days. It may seem now as though it was a steady upward progress, but in reality there were many times when I felt as though I had reached a plateau and couldn't break through to the next level. There were also times when I took a nosedive and had setbacks, and while sometimes it was the result of exceeding my limits, other times it was because I seemed to have picked up a virus, and sometimes I just couldn't find any reason - it just happened. This was one of the hardest things to cope with at the time.

Mental function also needed to be gradually rebuilt. It was progress when I began being able to watch "Countdown" every day, and I am not ashamed to say that the word and maths puzzles helped me to begin practicing being able to concentrate again. Gradually I was able to listen to the radio more during the day and then begin using the computer in my search for information which would help me to recover. I had to ration my computer sessions, but this was another great source of comfort and provided me with a sense of not being so isolated with this illness.

At a much later stage I began to see an osteopath. I read the book "The Back and Beyond" by Dr. Paul Sherwood and became interested in his theory that back problems leading to malfunctioning of the lymphatic system are a possible cause of Chronic Fatigue Syndrome. I also read about Raymond Perrin's work. He is an osteopath based in Stockport, who has treated many people with ME with some degree of success. I have continued to have cranial-sacral osteopathic treatment regularly, every four to six weeks, as I believe it helps me to stay well.

This led me later to seek the help of a lymphatic drainage massage therapist. I was at the point of being close to recovered but still not quite there. I found this therapy immediately and dramatically helpful. My brain fog improved markedly and energy levels were boosted. The drawback was that at £30 a time I could not afford more than a few weekly sessions, so I bought my own Chi Machine which has a similar effect. This was one of the final pieces in the jigsaw that enabled me to start living a normal life again.

A local ME support group gave me contact with others who had ME and that was literally a lifeline for me for a long time. I also took up singing. It was perfectly possible to sit down and sing if you needed to. In fact another woman with ME later joined who could not stand at all, and she was able to sing while lying down!

One of the hardest things about being so ill was the social isolation. I was very lucky to have my family around me but I lost touch with a lot of friends and acquaintances because I didn't have the energy to maintain contact. The friends who took the trouble to visit me when I was very ill were few, but I so appreciated their kindness that I still feel a close bond with those people to this day.

Recovery was a process which happened in stages over six years or so. For the first two years I was very ill, for another two I was moderately affected and for the last two years I remained too ill to take on paid work, but was gradually able to take on more commitments and to be more active. I gradually regained something like a normal social life. I could go to the theatre or cinema, meet a friend for coffee or go to someone's house for a meal or to the occasional party. I may have had to spend the day in bed to be able to manage it but while out I could appear fairly normal. I can remember the first time I was able to dance again, about four years on. I was over the moon.

I had always hoped I would be able to work again, though for a long time it seemed an impossible dream. I had no idea what sort of work I would be able to do if and when I got better. It took me over four years to get my NHS pension, but that meant I could never return to work as a Health Visitor or equivalent job in the NHS. One day I spotted an advertisement appealing for volunteers at a local Citizen's Advice Bureau. Within weeks I began as an administrative volunteer, with a commitment of three hours a week. After a few months I was improving so much that I dared to apply for training as an advice worker; a bigger commitment of one and a half days per week.

I was thrilled to have found such interesting work. I loved the job and my confidence increased tremendously. I continued as a volunteer advice worker for a year and then took the plunge into paid work, when I was certain that my improved health was more than a "blip". I was lucky enough to get a part-time post as a welfare rights adviser as my first step into paid work. This was a really important milestone for me. I absolutely love being able to make a real financial contribution again as well as being out in the world, meeting people, being useful and learning something new each day.

I now see myself as fully recovered from ME. Being well again has meant the world to me and I savour every day that I am able to be active all day long and simply do the things that most people take for granted. It is no problem for me now to walk the two miles or so to work, work an eight hour day, go home and make a meal for the family and then go out again in the evening. For many years that would have been beyond my wildest dreams!

On a personal level, I do feel that I have learned a great deal from the experience of serious illness, but at a high cost. It is not a journey I would wish on anyone else. I am a happier person now and have learned to take a very pragmatic approach to problems. I really appreciate every single day of wellness, knowing what the alternative could be. I am certainly much more at peace with myself and therefore with others too.

Most useful aid to recovery - Dr Sarah Myhill

Recommended books
"Recovering from ME" by Dr. William Collinge
"Treating Candida Through Diet" by Gill Jacobs
"The Back and Beyond" by Dr. Paul Sherwood

Recommended websites
www.drmyhill.com
www.merge.com
www.forme-cfs.co.uk
www.electronichealing.co.uk

Maggie Leathley

Jessica's Story

New found energy with Chinese herbs

Jessica was eleven years old in the year 2000 and she was a very active girl. She danced three times a week and played hockey for the school team. She played violin, piano and enjoyed singing lessons and she also performed in theatre and dancing shows and took part in musical competitions. During May 2000 Jessica caught a virus and after three or four weeks she returned to school, but she still didn't feel well.

At first we didn't know what was wrong with Jessica, we thought her lack of energy was connected with her growth rate as she was growing very quickly and suffered pain in her limbs and joints. She was a ballet dancer and had just started learning point work when, two weeks later, she had grown out of her ballet point shoes. She found she had no strength in her limbs and she was experiencing a great deal of pain. This included tummy pains which our doctor put down to bowel problems. Because Jessica is a vegetarian she may have been lacking in vitamins, minerals and fibre. Eventually Jessica became so ill that she could hardly move. She had to be helped to the toilet and she couldn't climb the stairs without assistance. She spent all her time sleeping, listening to music and watching Tom and Jerry cartoons on television - apparently the fast movement of cartoon characters keeps the brain active in conjunction with eye contact. She had neck and back problems and she ached all over. She experienced sweating attacks during the night, spasms in her legs and feet, and nightmares. She was also always cold, probably because her body wasn't producing any heat as she didn't move around very much.

Jessica's aunt, Juliet, suggested that Jessica's condition was post viral fatigue syndrome. She herself had been suffering from similar symptoms and had been researching on the internet and talking to her sister who is a doctor in the USA. We didn't want to accept Juliet's diagnosis because we knew how devastating this illness could be, so we asked our doctor for help. Unfortunately he couldn't give us any useful advice, but he did arrange for some blood tests thinking she may have glandular fever, but they came back negative. We have been told that ME can be brought on by a terrible shock. Well, in one year our family had experienced three separations and eventually all three parties had got divorced. This had had a devastating effect on Jessica because we were a very close family and we used to organise events and holidays together, and suddenly in a matter of years all these relationships had changed; I think Jessica found this very difficult to cope with.

So we continued life as best we could and Jessica would have good days and bad days. Many people didn't understand the illness. Even we as a family had terrible problems because Jessica's father and brother didn't believe there was anything wrong with her - they thought it was just a teenage problem and that she didn't want to go to school. But Jessica has always been a person who likes to be involved with everything, so why would she want to stay at home and not be with her friends and go to parties and take part in activities and music?

One day we were put in contact with a lady called Sue, who was wonderful with Jessica. Sue tried to explain to her that we can't control the decisions made by members of the family regarding their relationships and that we have to try to adapt to different situations. She also advised us to alter Jessica's diet because some of the foods she was eating were not suiting her body at that time. We established that we needed to omit certain foods such as potatoes, tomatoes, carrots, aubergines, peppers, cucumbers, chocolate and nuts. Dairy foods didn't agree with her either, and after trying various different types of milk, we found that she was happiest with rice milk. Water was her main source of liquid and we only gave her bottled water to drink and used bottled water to cook with. (Since making the change the family have noticed that we don't suffer with sore throats and colds, which had been a problem in the past. It may be a coincidence but we have been using bottled water ever since). We put Jessica onto organic foods as much as we could because we believed that she was sensitive to chemicals. We had the added complication of Jessica being a vegetarian and not even eating fish. We had her body PH balanced as she was still having problems with constipation and a lack of energy, and all these problems were thought to be a result of her diet.

Jessica wasn't improving enough with just the change in her diet, and so her singing teacher, who knew her very well, recommended acupuncture treatment. Her son, who was suffering with similar fatigue problems, had found that acupuncture treatment was very helpful. So naturally we started taking her for regular treatment. At first we couldn't believe the difference it made to her health. She began walking, she started smiling and she felt stronger again. We were so happy and she was able to return to school. However, she continued to have relapses and some days she would sleep from eight in the evening until midday the next day, or even later. She missed out in so many ways - she couldn't play her violin, and she had to stop her singing and dancing lessons - However, we continued with the acupuncture over the next eighteen months and it helped enormously, and by the summer of 2003 Jessica had started to stabilise and appeared to have stopped growing. She managed to attend a music course, and although she couldn't take part in everything and had to rest during the day, she managed to complete the week.

During the summer of the following year Jessica's health deteriorated and we got an appointment with a paediatrician. We had to wait several months for the appointment and so by the time we saw him she had recovered to a reasonable level. He told us that we were doing everything possible by controlling her life style and diet and that there was nothing more that could be done for her, although he did give us a letter confirming our diagnosis of chronic fatigue syndrome for school purposes. The paediatrician advised us that hopefully she would grow out of the symptoms, as indeed children are very likely to do.

When Jessica returned to school in the Autumn term 2004 she was looking and feeling very good. Unfortunately, she caught a virus and her health deteriorated again until she was so weak she didn't have the energy to talk. Her body shut down and all she wanted to do was sleep. Weeks went by and we were very worried about her health and mental state. At this time Jessica was unable to attend school at all and the pressure on us was immense. We were asked to report to the school each day on her progress and to confirm whether she was able to attend school or not. Bear in mind that she would sleep until twelve midday or two o'clock in the afternoon. She would go to bed at six thirty or seven o'clock in the evening, with bed socks and a hot water bottle, but would wake up in the night sweating and with pains in her legs and be unable to go back to sleep for a long time, so when I woke her in the morning at seven o'clock she would either not respond or groan asking why I was waking her up, because she felt so tired. The nightmare just didn't seem to stop.

At half term in October 2004 we invited a boy called Henry to come and stay a couple of days with us. It was arranged on the understanding that if Jessica didn't feel well we would cancel the arrangement. Jessica had met him when she had attended the summer music course at Haileybury. On the first day I took them to Longleat so they could see the animals from the car without having to do a great deal of walking, and it all went well. However, the next day Jessica was feeling very ill, aching all over, cold, crying and in a terrible state. On Henry's return to London he told his parents about Jessica's problems and they very kindly telephoned to tell us about Doctor Wang. They told us Dr Wang had helped many people with various medical problems and he had had remarkable success.

So the turning point in Jessica's life was when we contacted Doctor Wang and consequently visited his clinic in London. He actually told me that he could cure ME. Nobody had ever been able to say that to me before. We went to London and Jessica was given some acupuncture treatment, which was different from her previous treatments. He attached electrodes to the needles in her legs, which increased the power of the acupuncture. He then put very special long needles horizontally either side of her spine, about ten in total. Doctor Wang explained that he was treating the meridian points to stimulate her spleen, kidneys and liver, which weren't functioning correctly. She always suffered with neck problems and so he carried out treatment on her neck. Altogether the treatments took about one hour. Jessica never complained and she said it didn't hurt either. He then prescribed Chinese natural herb powders and herbal pills. Doctor Wang had a special recipe for his herbal medicines and they were carefully weighed. We had to mix two spoonfuls in luke warm water three times a day, half an hour before each meal. The herbs didn't taste very nice but, hey if they were going to make you better after years of feeling ill, wouldn't you try anything? Jessica got used to taking the herbs.

We were told the treatment would take about eight to ten weeks and that after that period she would still feel weak, as you do when you are recovering from an attack of flu. This may seem a long time to some people but when you have been ill for nearly four years it is no time at all. Doctor Wang changed the medicines slightly according to how Jessica felt each week. Of course my husband thought this was all a waste of time and money, driving up to London every week, but I believed in Doctor Wang and his recipe book of Chinese herbal medicines. It was very old and had been handed down to him. The Chinese have been treating people for thousands of years, so they must have learned something about medicine! Interestingly, Doctor Wang advised us that ME is a western medical problem as there are few cases in China.

The nearer we got to Christmas the greater Jessica's health improved. She was able to attend some days at school and she was sleeping much better. We decided as it was the Christmas holidays and New Year that we would leave her treatment for two weeks before we returned to

London for further acupuncture, but she would continue with the herbal medicines. We were delighted as Jessica was beginning to return to the daughter whom we had always known before her illness. We traveled to see Doctor Wang for a few more weekly visits and then we extended the visit to every two weeks and then we would visit every three weeks and then once a month and finally once in two months. During this period Jessica continued taking the herbs and eventually she stopped taking the herbs for one week and then re-introduced them for the next week and so on, but this wasn't for long.

By January 2005 the teachers couldn't believe the difference in Jessica. She was full of life and keen to learn and take part in so many school activities. We gradually re-introduced her to music and physical exercise. It was a miracle to see her enjoying herself and looking so happy.

By June 2005, Jessica was leading a fairly normal life. She hadn't missed any days at school and she was taking part in so many activities. She still felt tired if she pushed her body too much, but it was a different type of tiredness.

This year, in 2007, Jessica took up running – well, when you haven't been able to run for years I suppose it has it's attractions! Unknown to us, Jessica started training with her House Mistress and her school friends for a half-marathon! We couldn't believe that she could keep running for miles and miles. On the 1st May 2007 she completed the course and raised £260 for an African charity. As you can imagine, we are extremely proud of her!

In July she went to Italy with the school choir for ten days, and a few days later flew to Spain with friends. And in August she joined a week long music course with lots of rehearsals and concerts and then finally, she went to Sardinia for a rest. Jessica's recovery has enabled her to get her life back and enjoy the wonderful opportunities that come her way.

You may remember I mentioned Jessica's aunt, Juliet, who had very similar symptoms. By September 2006 she was struggling to walk and was unable to work. I was very concerned as Juliet is divorced and solely responsible for her two teenage children and if she was unable to work I dread to think what may have happened. So I offered to drive Juliet to London to be treated by Dr Wang, and, because she had seen the fantastic improvement in Jessica's health, she decided to take up my offer. So once again we traveled to London for treatment and, as before, we didn't see any huge improvement for a number of weeks, but gradually Juliet started to feel more human again. The cloudy brain and concentration span improved as did her physical body. Eventually, Juliet was strong enough to work from home and then she built up gradually over a period of a year to full time employment back at the office.

It was, and still is, so wonderful to see Jessica enjoying life and not suffering as she did for so many years. It is also wonderful for the family, as this kind of illness affects everyone. We would like to thank Nadine. Nadine has known Jessica since they were at infant school and they went dancing together and have always been close. Nadine would come and sit with Jessica when she was unable to do anything at all, and she knew not to talk but that just being there was a comfort to her. We can never thank Henry enough for introducing us to Doctor Wang, who has helped Jessica and our family so much. And of course our thanks to Dr Wang who has made all this possible with his treatments. We now have our daughter back and it is absolutely wonderful. Maybe Dr Wang can help you too!

Postscript by Jessica

My life is now fantastic

When I look back at how my life was, it was like I was disabled and couldn't do anything for myself. Climbing the stairs was like climbing Mount Everest! Teachers and friends at school thought I was faking it and not wanting to go to school but this just wasn't the case. I remember attending school, then getting so tired I had to lie on the sofa in the lounge and wait for my dad to take me home. I felt really lonely, especially when I had a boyfriend and couldn't see him for so long! Texting and phone calling was the only way of contact.

During my recovery I was able to go out with my friends but I was scared in case of a relapse, so I had to try and understand not to do too much at once. These days I don't have to be so cautious and I am enjoying life as a result.

Being cured in just eight months has changed my life dramatically. I can now sprint a football pitch and I have run a half marathon. Achieving something so immense feels great. The reason for me wanting to put myself up for such a challenge is because I needed to boost my confidence again. During the period of not being able to move or do much exercise my weight increased and I looked like a balloon. I also found it hard to perform because I didn't feel good about my appearance, which made me more nervous, and I ended up being disappointed and depressed because I had lost my talent to perform. My focus has now changed and I have experimented with foods and made my diet healthier, increased my exercise by running more and this is what helped me get back into shape.

I can attend academic lessons and not feel sleepy but I do get the occasion of wanting to fall asleep because of an un-enthusiastic teacher! One problem that remains is my memory. I sometimes find it difficult to remember things and I have overcome this by having a busy schedule. I am much more organised and I think better.

Dr Wang is wonderful, kind and caring, a great cook and a dedicated man to helping those with medical problems. If it wasn't for him and his medical expertise I wouldn't of been able to full fill my dreams of singing and dancing and now that I am fully recovered I can now focus and make those dreams come true. I shall always be grateful to him for the rest of my life.

Most useful aid to recovery - Dr Y J Wang, Portland Close, Edmunton, London N9 0XN
Tel No. 020 8345 6261 Mobile No. 07958 207 193

Rosalind and Jessica's advice - we feel that Chinese herbs and eventually regular exercise builds up the strength of the body and that a good diet is important.

Rosalind and Jessica Crabtree

Christine's Story

To start my recovery I had to slow down

I will start by telling you a wee bit about myself. I am fifty-six years old, small, petite with a bubbly personality and I moved to Essex from Scotland, with my two sons, over eighteen years ago to work full time in Southend. I did this because most of my brothers and my sister have lived in England for the last twenty-odd years and I wanted to be closer to them. I made lots of new friends and many have remained so to this date. Before I was ill I enjoyed a good social life with my husband going to the gym, walking, badminton, dancing, shopping, driving, cinema and sometimes a barn dance.

In September 1996 at work, there were a lot of colds and flu about the time I started to feel unwell. I just gradually began to feel tired. I used to go to the works' gym twice a week on my lunch break. At first I just got awfully tired walking back up the stairs to my desk and I thought I was overdoing it, so I got the lift instead. But that didn't seem to help. Then I thought I needed to eat lunch first for more energy, but that didn't work either, and I still felt awfully tired. So I decided to drop a day and only go once a week. That didn't help either! Eventually I had to cut out the gym altogether, which was a shame as I really enjoyed it.

I couldn't understand what was wrong with me. I was so tired all the time, no energy, not sleeping well at night. Some nights I would be so tired I would go to bed straight after my evening meal at 7pm, when I would toss and turn all night and would wake up in the morning still feeling exhausted.

As the months passed my colleagues would often ask if I was all right. I would say I was fine but they could see that I wasn't. My walking club was only once a month so I kept doing it for as long as I could. The walks varied from four to eight miles, so I just went on the shorter walks and missed out on the longer ones, but after three months I had to give that up as well. By now I had no energy to do anything other than work. Everything was suffering. I could not do any housework or shopping and even thinking what to cook for dinner at night was hard work. The funny thing is that I even found chewing my food exhausting!

Everything I did outside of work stopped, even meeting with friends. I used to come in from work and get into a bath where I would try and feel better. It was like I was on a merry-go-round, and it was going round and round and I couldn't stop it. This was a very difficult time for my husband and family as they couldn't understand what was wrong with me. I was constantly in a bad mood and lost my temper all the time. I often said to him that it was no fun being married to me, as all I did was sleep and moan.

I was struggling to complete a full day at work. I had flexi-working hours, which was lucky in that I could leave work earlier than normal. I started getting terrible headaches all the time and I would swallow paracetamol every four hours. My eyes had trouble focusing and everything seemed to get blurred. I used to blame it on the lighting at work. I didn't go to the doctor. As I couldn't describe what was wrong with me how could I explain it to him? I just felt awful all the time, exhausted and headachy. I got a pair of glasses to see if that would take the headaches away, but they didn't. I had aching limbs, eyes not focusing, no concentration and a foggy brain. It was a constant struggle to get myself to work every day. It got so bad that one day I arrived at work and couldn't take off my coat. I just laid my head on my arms on the desk and told my colleagues that I would be OK in a

few minutes. They threatened to call the doctor themselves
make an appointment. So I did.

I went to my doctor that morning – 4 March 1997. I tried to
explain what I felt like. He sent me for blood tests and they all came
back normal. I was off work sick for eight weeks. On my sick certificate
it said 'viral infection'. After the eight weeks I felt slightly better and
my doctor suggested I return to work. I trusted him completely, but
on hindsight this was the wrong thing to do.

I returned to work slowly by doing a few hours a day and a few
days a week, until I was working full time again, which took roughly a
month. For the next three years I worked and slept, worked and slept,
worked and slept – and did nothing else. I had no social life, I had no
energy for it. I gave up everything so I would have enough energy to
go to work and hope to do a full week, going to bed at 7pm until 7am
every single night and still waking up un-refreshed. In time I no longer
had enough energy to do even one day a week at work. I would spend
the rest of the week off sick and even after that I still felt exhausted
the following week. It was just like having a bad dose of the flu all the
time. Even walking jarred my whole body.

Eventually I saw a consultant in December 1999 who diagnosed
me with ME/CFS. He told me that there was no one he could send me
to who could make me better. I felt I couldn't carry on the way I was.
There must be someone who could help me. So a friend of a friend
found a doctor, Dr David Smith, who specialised in the diagnosis,
management and treatment of ME.

My first appointment was in May 2000. It was the most emotional
and wonderful day of my life, as Dr Smith actually listened to me and
understood what I was saying. He didn't make me feel that all I had
suffered these last three years was just in my mind. There was a promise
that I could get better with this treatment of an activity programme
and medication. It terrified me at first that it would take roughly four
to five years. It seemed an awfully long time to be on this medication,
but Dr Smith explained that it would take this long because of my
age and how long I had been ill. At first I wasn't sure about the whole

treatment, but I felt I had no choice if I wanted to get better. After-all, there was no-one else out there that wanted to help me!

Dr Smith advised me to give up work so together my husband and I had to make the decision for me to retire from work. I was very lucky to have the support of a lovely husband and family, because things got very difficult for us when I was very ill and it took them a long time to understand how ill I was. Without my money coming in things would get very difficult financially for us.

To start my recovery I had to slow everything down and just do five minute tasks with rest breaks and move forward very slowly. The most difficult thing I found to slow down was my brain. It would not rest at all. What helped a bit was to meditate, which took a wee while to master. I found the strict activity programme along with various medications hard to get into and it took nearly eighteen months to get the hang of it. I had to sit down to do things like ironing or peeling potatoes. I would see Dr Smith every four to six weeks when he would help move me forward slowly. Every year I would see a slight improvement in what I could do. Simple things like hanging out a whole line of washing, or hovering one room. So over the years I was able to do my housework without feeling tired. It took five years of moving very slowly until I got better. I gave myself some goals. I learned to swim, which also relaxes me, and I walk every day. Mentally my emotions are still delicate. I get upset very easily with arguments.

I would love to say a big thank you to Dr Smith. He gave me back my life by his undivided support, patience and full commitment to me. Thank you also to my husband, family and friends who were there for me when I needed them.

Most useful aid to recovery - Dr David Smith

Recommended website - www.me-cfs-treatment.com

Christine's advice - I would like to say to anyone reading my story to get help as early as possible, because I pushed myself much too hard trying to put mind over matter. It took me a long, long time to change my life around, because that's what I had to do in order to get my life back.

Christine Patient

Diana's Story

Healing layer by layer - my walk with CFS

For most of my life (read before CFS) I'd been known as a particularly festive, high-energy person. In my adolescent years people would often remark, "I want what she's on." I was high on nothing save life, and its run-of-the-mill vicissitudes notwithstanding, was good.

The irony of course was that when CFS came creeping, and then storming, into my life, I became the polar opposite - a broken, brittle, lifeless, empty shell - I was gone. And I wept in raw self-pity at the grave of the self I felt I'd lost forever.

It all started in my mid-thirties when I stopped nursing my then one-year-old son. I was sad to give up the closeness with him, but it was time and I was looking forward to getting my body back. But the body I got back was not my pre-pregnancy body, and I'm not talking stretch marks here, or a less-than-pancake-flat tummy, what I was about to deal with had nothing to do with body image, and everything to do with a body broken.

The downward spiral started unremarkably enough with a general feeling of weakness and malaise. Next, came an endless stream of sinus infections. No stamina. No defences. Unrelenting fatigue and body aches. I began calling myself "The Girl in the Plastic Bubble." My regular doctor pooh-poohed my tail of woe and told me that it was not uncommon for young mothers to catch viruses from their babies and have more of them than the "average bear." (Yogi Bear).

My family also seemed complacent with my then functional sickness, that is, until I announced one day that I was dying and that when I fell asleep I felt as if I were sinking into the earth's core, and that one day I might never wake up. Then they rallied. I went to see a Harvard-educated immunologist referred by a family friend. This doctor did a battery of tests and diagnosed me with Common Variable Immune Deficiency (CVID) an immune disorder one has from birth but which manifests in the third or fourth decade of life. His treatment was IVIG – intravenous immuno-gamma globulin. I tried the monthly infusion twice, but got no relief. By now I was experiencing violent viruses with high fevers, and for all intents and purposes, was bedridden.

I decided to get a second opinion. I chose a holistic doctor who came highly-recommended and for whom there was a waiting list to become a patient. I have now been seeing this doctor for more than four years and have undertaken a variety of treatments. Her diagnosis was Epstein-Barr/CFS. Over time and with Dr. Watson's help I was able to get out of bed and begin a life of low-level functioning. She helped me change my diet and put me on a regimen of herbs and nutritional supplements. I, in turn, sought counselling, read books on health and healing, joined the CFS Association of America, began a serious meditation practice and surfed the internet looking for clues, and cures, for my health challenges. Dr. Watson also began work on my endocrine system, as she'd found my hormone levels to be completely out of whack and I began to supplement with natural testosterone and later, progesterone.

As time went by there were good days. However, pacing myself, taking time to rest and managing my severe hypoglycaemia and nocturnal eating issues, became an integral part of my daily existence. Of course, the good days seemed all too few, interrupted as they were by regular bouts of illness and often depression. One day, during my daily meditation, I 'saw' my illness as an onion; I was peeling away layer after paper-thin layer of dysfunction, but it was slow going, and there were so many more layers to go.

And so the years of battling my illness went by, counted by how old my son was minus one. Haunting my husband and me during my walk with CFS was our desire for another child, a sibling for our little boy. We watched the months slip by and turn into years. We were uncertain whether I could handle a pregnancy, let alone care for another life. When I brought it up with my doctor she would always respond in the same way, "Why don't we wait another six months?" Meanwhile, I wasn't getting any younger.

On Easter Morning, 2004, we threw caution to the wind and were stunned a few weeks later when we learned I had conceived. I called it our miracle baby. What followed was three months of nausea and vomiting – a mirror image of my first pregnancy. However, what I felt building under the pregnancy sickness was yet another miracle - stamina, strength and the long sought-after health.

Tragedy struck at my three-month check-up. There was no heartbeat. Our miracle baby had died. Nothing had prepared us for the loss of the baby we had prayed and longed for. We were devastated. Calls, cards, emails and visits from friends and family comforted us in our grief, but did not take away the emptiness and the aching to see and hold our baby. As my body became 'not pregnant' what I had sensed was there, underneath the unpleasant symptoms of the first trimester, began to manifest. I revelled in my newfound strength and praised God for the miracle of a functioning body. Further research into the matter found anecdotal evidence that, in some cases, illness brought on by pregnancy could be healed by it. I believed it was true.

And so that summer turned to fall and I braced myself for the cold and flu season, telling myself that this time I would not be taken down by colds, flu and other viruses, because being pregnant had reset my hormones and healed my embattled immune system. However, what I did not realize was that there was one more layer to go in my path to total wellness. Indeed, as the thermostat dropped, my achilles heel began to rear its nasty head. I began to fall ill with sinus infection after sinus infection, a pattern that had played a big part in the on-set of my CFS back in 2001. However, this time things were different I told myself. I not only had my endocrine system under control, but gone was the unrelenting fatigue and the rest of the debilitating symptoms that characterize CFS. Still, when I could barely manage to stay well for even a week before getting another, or the same, sinus infection, and when the doctors started doling out fourteen-day courses of antibiotics instead of ten, I began to fear I was going back into "the dark hole."

I meditated, I prayed for help - and it came, in the form of a CT-scan, which showed blockages, polyps, and mucous retention cysts in my maxillary and ethmoid sinuses. An ENT specialist suggested surgery. I was unsure until I meditated on it and heard "have the surgery" so forcefully in my head that it was almost as if the words had been uttered. In May 2005 I underwent endoscopic sinus surgery at UCLA Medical Center and have never looked back. My walk with CFS had ended.

Currently, my husband and I are in the midst of adoption proceedings. I feel strong, ready and capable of caring for another life. However, I have chosen not to become pregnant myself, careful and cautious as I am to protect my body, my onion – peeled back as it has been, to its inner and most radiant core.

Most useful aid to recovery - ENT surgery

Recommended books
"Adrenal Fatigue: The 21st Century Stress Syndrome" by James L. Wilson
"The Low Blood Sugar Handbook" by Edward & Patricia Kimmel
"Prescription to Nutritional Healing" by Phyllis A. Balch
"Spiritual Survival Guide: How to Find God When You're Sick" by Dr.Charles Shields
"There's a Spiritual Solution to Every Problem" by Dr. Wayne Dyer

Recommended websites
www.cfids.org
www.webMD.com
www.annahemmings.com

Medical Referral - Dr. Cynthia Watson, Santa Monica, CA   Tel: 310 315-9101

Diana's advice - believe you can heal yourself, that within you resides the power to heal. Ask questions. Contact local support groups, write healing affirmations and post them by your bed, meditate, listen to and observe your body, celebrate improvements, pray.

Diana Foutz Daniele

Ute's Story

I always knew there would be light at the end of the tunnel

I had ME in 1989/90 and my doctor never really figured out at the time what my mysterious illness was. I was being checked out for glandular fever, multiple sclerosis, a heart condition, arthritis and cancer amongst other things and I'm sure the medics thought of me as a hypochondriac.

It had all started with me being bedridden after having suffered a flu type illness that I just couldn't shake off. What incapacitated me most was physical weakness and constant pain in all my muscles, especially in the legs. At my worst I couldn't even lift my arms above my head. I felt like a zombie as a result of insomnia, despite feeling extremely fatigued all the time. Looking after three small children became practically impossible and I needed help in more ways than one.

A couple of months into the illness I struck lucky. My husband discovered a neighbour and the wife of an acquaintance with similar symptoms, who were healing themselves with the help of a very strict candida diet. From the moment I went on this diet I felt as if I was taking control again. It took me several months to gain enough energy to walk up or down the stairs more than once a day, and a few more before I ventured out on tiny shopping trips accompanied by my very supportive husband. He was happy to ferry me and the kids around as it meant a stimulating break for everyone.

However a smooth progressive recovery it wasn't! About six months into my illness my GP referred me to a heart specialist who was looking for guinea pigs to try a controversial sleep cure. I agreed to being sedated for a week as I was desperate to get better faster if I could. However I hadn't been warned that I could become addicted to Valium and other sedatives. Weaning myself off them took me months, during which I found myself in a constant state of anxiety. The 'cure' had also turned out to be a curse for many other sufferers, as I discovered later.

During this time I felt as if I was starting over from scratch. Although I wasn't feeling depressed I agreed to take a six month course of antidepressants. Thankfully they helped me to sleep better and gradually made me feel better physically. I kept the candida diet going throughout, consulted an excellent homeopath and supplemented with courses of Echinacea and large doses of Vitamins. What also helped me was to rest or sleep twice a day at the same time as my kids, eventually cutting the breaks down to a siesta after lunch to recharge my batteries. I made a point of learning to read my body's signals very carefully and only ever did physically what my body told me it could cope with. As a result my recovery seemed like one step forward at a time ,but with the occasional step back. Eighteen months later I'd dropped down two dress sizes and looked rather worse for wear, but I could tell that I was on the mend. Not long after that I was ready to join the gentlest of yoga classes that I could find.

A few years later my doctor asked me whether I had fully recovered. I had, especially mentally. On a physical level I never quite managed to achieve a level of fitness comparable to someone who has never had ME, but I was no Lance Armstrong and so it wasn't a problem. What helped me though the worst of my ME times was my unshaken belief that ME was not at all in the mind but in my body, like an extended flu that would eventually get better. I had suffered a lot of stress in the year before I became ill, and felt that my immune system must have been quite suppressed.

My biggest learning was not to fight ME but to accept it and go with it and to learn to be patient. I always knew there would be light at the end of the tunnel ... as indeed there was ...

Most useful aid to recovery - anti-candida diet

Recommended website - www.afme.co.uk

Ute Wieczorek-King

Norah's Story

Take Control of your life

Chronic fatigue syndrome and fibromyalgia have been a long, difficult and expensive road for me.

The only prescription medications I took were Tylenol and Flexoril, so I didn't have much medical support. I took my healthcare into my own hands and tried all of the following: acupuncture, massage therapy, a chiropractor, physiotherapy, osteopathy, holistic nutrition, mega supplements, workouts at the gym with a personal trainer and pool therapy. It was a full-time job!

Two years ago I took my summer vacation in a wheelchair. Last year I started studying alternative medicine. Exams, homework, projects and studying have completely taken over my life. In a year I went from having difficulties getting out of bed, to studying full-time again. I would never have believed that I could go back to school and learn a new career let alone be at the top of my class! I've been doing so well both with my health and in school that the massage therapist has committed to hiring me as a reflexologist and clinical aromatherapist when I graduate. Two years ago I would have never believed all this could happen to me, but it has!

I believe that anyone can go into remission if they want to badly enough. There isn't anything the human body can't heal itself from, including cancer.

The only way healing can be done with alternative medicine is to be committed no matter how difficult. Change your diet with whole foods; do the exercises no matter how inconvenient; change the personal attitude – put self pity where it belongs and take control of your life!

What did I find most useful? Massage therapy, acupuncture, osteopathy, reflexology, holistic nutrition, organic foods, eliminating red meat and dairy, increasing the correct vegetables, swimming, walking the treadmill, using a core stability ball … all these things and no one thing was the answer. They all complimented each other.

I went from being wheelchair-bound to studying alternative medicine so that I can help those who want to help themselves, instead of relying on traditional medicine to give them a miracle fix. I may sound harsh, but these are the facts. So many people sit back, whine and cry, pop the pills and won't fight the good fight. I reached the bottom of the pit, yelled out to my higher power … "either I die now, or I find a way to get healthy, but this is not life".

I looked for life, fought hard for it, and found it. I hope you do too.

Recommended website - www.wholehealth.com This website was a great help. Here I found out about calcium/magnesium and my life-saver – 5-HTP.

Norah Bleazard

Naomi's Story

God was always there

We spent seven years in Zambia where my husband was the doctor in a bush mission hospital. I looked after our two sons and helped out where I could. While I was there I caught malaria and had lots of dysentery problems which weakened my body.

In 1993 we returned to England, but unfortunately my health didn't pick up. I was in the boom and bust stage. In January 1997 I caught a virus and went downhill from then on. We knew I had to slow down but I didn't realise I was still pushing myself so much.

In November 1998 I went on a Westcare residential week (now run by Action for ME) and that was the turning point. For the first time I really stopped. I paced myself as well as I could with a family to look after. It was about a year before I saw improvement and then it was two steps forward and one back.

Meanwhile I had investigations for continuing gut problems. Three months of antibiotics and an exclusion diet on the advise of a dietician trained in allergies. I removed all dairy products and that did bring some improvement. As did acupuncture, until the GP who was doing it became ill.

Looking back I made very slow progress, with many setbacks, from being housebound with a downstairs bedroom as I was unable to climb stairs, to having a wheelchair when outside.

It was my Christian faith that gave me strength through the long dark days. God was always there. I could scream and shout at him but he never stopped loving me and giving me encouragement. Screaming at God also meant I was less likely to shout at the family!

Eventually I became more independent, especially when both my lads were at university. Shopping on my own was great, as was sending the wheelchair back. My husband was asked if I had died when he phoned to ask them to take it away!

My gut problems were still not completely better so in September 2004 we went to the Centre for Complimentary Medicine in Southampton. The doctor there thought I still had tropical bugs in my gut and still some of the virus that had triggered the crisis. The homeopathic medicine made me feel worse at first but after that my recovery speeded up. He also gave me Active Life, a vitamin and mineral supplement that is absorbed at the top of the gut and so avoiding the damage.

I was still left with brain fog, though it didn't stop me having five extra people staying over Christmas, followed by my mother's 80th birthday in January. Yes it did knock me back, but recovery was so much quicker this time.

In February I went to a retired physiotherapist as I was having problems with my hip. After he had sorted that out I volunteered to try the Bowen Technique which he was now practicing. At the first session he said that my body was out of balance. It is a very gentle therapy, done through light clothing, so no tiring undressing. After four sessions the brain fog was improving and I haven't needed to return for more since. As always I know that it is God who ultimately does the healing, but he uses many different people and therapies.

Since then our oldest son has got engaged, my father in law has gone to be with his heavenly father and we went to London to celebrate an aunt's Golden wedding.

In July 2006 we celebrated our silver wedding with a meal for family and friends travelling a distance; followed by a thanksgiving during which we highlighted how God had helped us during our 25 years. We interspersed the chat with hymns and prayer and for this we were joined by folk from our Church. All those with enough energy completed the time with a Barn Dance. It was thrilling to be able to keep going all day, chatting, dancing and singing. It is so encouraging that, although tired the next day, I did not crash!

In between times I have been teaching relaxation with Christian meditations. When I was on the Action for ME's residential week we had relaxation and meditation and I was concerned about opening my mind to unhelpful things. God spoke to me and told me He would use it to strengthen my walk with Him and also to help others.

I have now recorded a CD of four exercises. The first is just relaxation. The other three are journeys to heaven, based on the end of the book of Revelation. If you are interested please contact me. (See below).

I am so thankful to God for the healing I have and I look to Him to see where He will lead me next.

Most useful aid to recovery - Christian faith

Recommended websites
www.afme.com
www.thebowentechnique.com
www.jonc.me.uk/relax

Naomi's advice - I recommend the Action for M.E. Residential Course

Naomi Cooper

Emma's Story

I became very creative in the kitchen

I was diagnosed with Chronic Fatigue Syndrome in June 1998. At the time I was at studying at university, plus working morning and night teaching aerobics, and training for competition aerobics every day. I also had an active social life. Having had glandular fever five years before, I was probably overdoing it.

I was diagnosed with CFS after seven months of severe weight loss and fatigue and various other debilitating symptoms including headaches, blurred vision, memory loss, inability to sleep and chronic bowel and stomach irritations. This diagnosis came from a wonderful doctor who I still see regularly today. He was the only doctor not to diagnose me with an eating disorder or a mental illness.

My weight plummeted from an athletic 58kg to a frightening 32kg in the space of about nine months. It seemed that the more food I ate the more weight I lost. Taking a gamble, my doctor sent me off to the Food Allergy Clinic at the Royal Prince Alfred Hospital Allergy Unit in Sydney, and we found what was to be the turning point in my battle with CFS. I was extremely sensitive to chemicals, both natural and artificial, in foods and perfumed products.

I was put on an extremely restricted diet of boiled white rice and white fish and within days many of my symptoms had begun to disappear. I no longer suffered from stomach pains and wind and my mouth ulcers were reduced in number. For someone who loves cooking and food this was very difficult to come to terms with, but since I was facing death if I kept going as I was, I was willing to give anything a go and stick to it rigidly. The side effects of not being disciplined were too great and the consequences too risky.

So I followed the chemical free diet, and within one month I had started to regain weight. It took about four months before I could start introducing the most basic of items such as green beans or potatoes and it didn't take much to tip me over the edge, but using the time I had (lots of it) I became very creative in the kitchen.

Within six months we could all see that this diet and way of life was the way in which I would fully recover.

I am now fortunate enough to eat whatever I like whenever I like. The turning point for me was my first pregnancy in 2003-2004. My body seemed to go back to normal in terms of tolerating a wide variety of foods. I still exclude wheat entirely from my diet, and if I am feeling run down or tired I go back to a very basic diet, as that is what my body seems to require, and it speeds up the recovery process. It is now just a case of common sense prevailing and me being in tune with my body and its needs.

I am now happily married with a beautiful two-year-old son, and I feel fantastic. I have recently sold a business which I started in 2000 to become a full time mother and help my husband out with some of our other business interests. It helps to have a focus and a goal such as a home-based business when recovering from any illness. It allows you to set some goals but gives you a degree of flexibility also.

I have experienced so much with my illness, but I am actually glad it happened to me. So many good things have come into my life because of CFS. My close relationships are even closer and I have a greater appreciation for the simple things in life and what it means to be able to get out of bed in the morning. I can now use my experiences to help others who have CFS and help to promote a very misunderstood and still poorly accepted illness.

Most useful aid to recovery - a chemical-free diet

Recommended websites
www.cs.nsw.gov.au
www.fedupwithfoodadditives.info

Emma

David's Story

I'm healthier and happier than I was before I got ill

It was December 2000, near the end of a two-week Christmas break, that my illness began. It started off with typical flu symptoms, sneezing and a runny nose, with the fever symptoms of feeling cold and aches and pains all over my body. After a few days the fever lifted, but I still felt tired and weak and had no appetite, so I assumed it would just take a few more days for my body to recover.

After about a week of this, still no sign of recovery and having to spend most of the day lying on the sofa, I went to see the doctor. I was told the usual "it's a virus, it can take up to ten days to recover" line. I accepted this, although it seemed a bit strange that I had virtually no appetite, even though I didn't have a fever any more. It certainly didn't seem like any flu I had had before. I was also mildly depressed for no apparent reason, which I assumed must have been another symptom.

About two weeks after the initial flu infection I started to feel gradually better but I discovered that if I tried to do too much I would regret it the next day. One day I woke up feeling energetic and decided to go for a run around the local park. The next day I woke up feeling barely alive and had to spend most of the day lying on the sofa again.

During this period I often didn't feel like eating anything until lunchtime, when I could manage soup and a piece of toast. I would then feel dead for most of the rest of the day until late afternoon, when

I had more energy and could manage to eat a normal meal. I found that if I ate too much at night I would have difficulty sleeping and I would end up awake for most of the night while my body struggled to digest. When this happened I would feel very weak again the next day.

I assumed that I just needed to give my body time to recover so I tried not to push my body too far until it was fully recovered.

About three or four weeks after the initial infection, I was feeling well enough to go back to work again. This resulted in a setback, with me feeling very weak and lacking in appetite for most of the time. However, as I wasn't doing anything particularly challenging in the job, it wasn't too much of a problem. I was working as an IT contractor, but this particular job just involved updating the occasional website and sitting around doing nothing for the rest of the time.

I arranged another doctor's appointment to figure out what was wrong with me. Post-viral fatigue was mentioned and I was told that most people eventually recover. The doctor asked about my lifestyle – was I getting enough exercise and did I have a good diet? Both of which I thought were fine. The doctor also asked about my job – was it too stressful? Was I worried about lack of money if I took time off sick? I pointed out that I had got sick after two weeks of holiday, that my job wasn't particularly stressful and that I had enough money in the bank to go for a year or two without working.

For the next three months my illness kept relapsing and remitting. I would usually go about a week feeling mostly okay, then for another week or so I would feel terrible. I would often have to take a day or two off work during the relapses and would then return to work.

As I continued to work, things started to get worse. I would take a few days off work and then return when I felt better. But instead of feeling okay for a week or two, I could now only manage a day or two back at work before the symptoms came back. I was also suffering from chronic insomnia and severe depression and anxiety during my bad periods. I had nothing on my mind and didn't have any reason to feel depressed, so I assumed they were symptoms. I also seemed to have a desynchronised body clock, sometimes feeling wide awake during the night and sleepy during the day. When this happened I would feel really tired and weak the next day and the depression would be a lot worse.

One day, after not being able to sleep all night for no apparent reason, I had acute depression the next day (9.5 on a scale of one to ten), followed by intense anxiety, followed by depression again, then anxiety in roughly one-hour cycles. The problem was clearly something in my brain – lack of neurotransmitters or a messed-up body clock – but it was confusing and frightening because I didn't know what was causing it or how to cure it. My doctor kept saying it was my lifestyle/job that was causing the problems, although I didn't see how that could be the case because my job wasn't very stressful. I pointed out to the doctor that my problem appeared to be a lack of stress tolerance rather than too much stress, but this distinction didn't seem significant to her.

Because my symptoms always improved when I took time off, I eventually decided to give up my job. Another person working with me told me that his wife had had a similar illness. She had kept taking sick days and going back to work again, and eventually she had developed ME and now couldn't work. I didn't want to end up in the same situation, so I decided that the best course of action would be to take a long break and sort myself out. The fact that I had depression was also a critical factor: the physical symptoms I could have coped with and dragged myself into work most days, but the depression was so severe that it forced me to actually do something about my situation as I simply couldn't continue any longer.

After leaving my job I recovered quickly and a month or so later I was feeling pretty much normal again. I made other changes to my life, such as moving away from London and moving in with my girlfriend, as well as spending more time working on my own projects and building up my own business. I was able to live a normal life and eventually went back to working on contracts again, but taking things sensibly and not wearing myself out.

Things went well until 2001 when I had a bad relapse in March and another one in July. During the second relapse I went to see another doctor. The worst of my symptoms at this time were lack of appetite, diarrhoea and insomnia. I asked the doctor if I could have a food allergy, as I seemed to have diarrhoea after eating certain foods, but she ruled this out and diagnosed irritable bowel syndrome. I mentioned to the doctor that I had been trying to make my life as stress-free as possible but I was still having symptoms. She pointed out that "some people need motivating activities" in their lives to feel normal. At the time this seemed a pretty stupid thing to say – did I need more stress in my life to feel normal? But it stuck in my mind, and only later did I realise the significance.

I was now spending a lot of time doing research into chronic fatigue syndrome, irritable bowel syndrome, stress, burnout and related areas such as the circadian body clock. All these areas seemed to be involved in the illness but I didn't know how it all fitted together. An important part seemed to be stress and stress tolerance. CFS seemed to be caused by an inability to *handle* stress, rather than simply too much stress.

Hans Selye pioneered stress research during the first half of the 20th century when he mapped out the body's response to stress. According to Selye there are three stages to the stress response: 1). the alarm stage, when the adrenal glands discharge all of their stored stress hormones into the blood. 2). the resistance stage, when the adrenal glands increase in size in order to maintain a high output of stress hormones. 3). the stage of exhaustion, which eventually comes after continued stress and results in symptoms similar to the alarm phase. During this phase the adrenal glands shrink and levels of cortisol fall, resulting in an inability to cope with stress.

CFS seemed to equate to Selyes' exhaustion stage. Low cortisol is a central feature of CFS with many studies showing that CFS patients have low cortisol, and in some cases highly shrunken adrenal glands.

It wasn't until January 2002 that I finally put all of the pieces together and realised what had caused my illness. The key was realising that my initial illness and subsequent relapses had all happened during times when I didn't have any work to do, usually after a period of hard work. The illness seemed to be caused by a combination of stress and lack of motivation and goals and simply reducing stress alone did not result in recovery. What did seem to help was having motivating, enjoyable activities.

Many people have reported that they initially contracted the illness when they have excessive responsibilities, or when they have multiple work and personal stressors from which there appears to be no way out. In my case I had been working on a full-time and part-time contract job as well as working on my own business. At the time I got ill I had just reduced my workload a lot and I wasn't particularly motivated by my work. I also had a number of minor interpersonal emotional issues, which caused a lot of pent-up anger and frustration. None of these factors alone was particularly significant and I didn't have any major psychiatric issues, a psychiatrist would presumably have given me a clean bill of health. It was the combination of a number of stressors, together with a lack of goals and motivation and a feeling that there was no way out, that caused my illness. After developing CFS, simply removing the stresses wasn't enough to recover, the illness puts the body into a state that is difficult to break out of and a positive effort is required to fully recover.

CFS and depression seem to be the body's way of telling you to change your lifestyle and the longer you try to avoid the message, the worse it will get. In my case I made significant changes relatively quickly, so I found it easier to recover than some other people I have spoken to.

Since realising the factors that caused my illness and what keeps me healthy, I have been in perfect physical and mental health for five years. Since my recovery, I usually walk or cycle for at least an hour a day and I have recently re-validated my private pilot's licence after a long period of not flying. I run my own business developing internet software. It is challenging and fun and I can decide when and what I work on. Since recovering I have got married and moved from the UK to Canada, both of which caused a lot of worry and stress, but no symptoms.

Although it might sound strange, the illness has actually improved my life and I am now much healthier and happier than I ever was before my illness!

Most useful aid to recovery - understanding the causes of the illness

Recommended books
"Flow: The Psychology of Optimal Experience" by Mihaly Csikszentmihalyi
"Chronic Fatigue Syndrome (CFS/ME): The Facts" by Frankie Campling & Michael Sharpe

Recommended websites
www.me-cfs-treatment.com
www.me-cfs-recovery.co.uk

Davids' advice - if I could give one piece of advice to anyone who thinks they may be contracting CFS it would be to make significant changes to your lifestyle at the earliest possible opportunity. It may be difficult, but you'll appreciate it in the long-run! It's also important to remember that people can and do make full recoveries from chronic and severe CFS and are able to live full and normal lives afterwards. Yes, recovery takes time and effort, but if you remove any negative stressors from your life and then work at slowly but gradually building up your mental and physical activity levels, then you stand a good chance of progressing towards recovery. Talk to other people who have recovered and see what works for them, but above all don't give up and never think that you will be ill for life - as that can be a self-fulfilling prophecy.

David Jameson

Rita's Story

The body, in its wisdom, takes over

It was my third year at the racetrack when the fatigue first set in. I was working in a very demanding job on the racecourses throughout the North of Britain. The job entailed driving a van with up to twelve staff to different racing venues each day. It was a highly pressurised job with a great deal of responsibility and some days I wouldn't arrive home until 10 pm at night. I lived alone, had little time for friends or leisure and it had been literally all bed and work for about two years. I had grown to hate the job and I felt over-worked and totally trapped.

The years prior to getting this job had been very unhappy for me. A divorce in 1977 meant I had had to move into a back-to-back house in an area which I found depressing. I had no support from my family and felt very lonely. The only light in my life was a very low-paid job, but I was happy there. Unfortunately I was made redundant. I quickly acquired another job and three months later was made redundant again. This led to a long spell of unemployment and after a while I was being treated for depression. In 1981 I was offered the job at the race-track.

In 1983 I felt unusually tired every morning and had no energy after work. Over a couple of months the fatigue worsened, with increasing muscle weakness and a feeling of just wanting to lie

290

down and sleep all the time. I was in so much pain in my neck, back, shoulders and arms that I just could not wait to finish work every night and get home.

There were occasions I remember when I would arrive home from work at teatime and wake up at 9 or 10 pm, with my untouched cup of tea on the coffee table and my jacket still on - I had literally fallen asleep as soon as I had sat down. On these occasions I would feel strangely disoriented on waking, like waking up from a coma, as if what I had done that day was all a dream. The muscular pain had gradually become unbearable and when I began to experience an uncontrollable urge to fall asleep at the wheel I had no choice but to give in and go on the sick. My 'autopilot' must have gone out then and I spent every day sleeping until dinner time, waking up feeling drugged and dazed, with every part of my body hurting. I was utterly mystified as to what was happening to me, and so were the doctors. Numerous tests from my doctor (GP) all proved negative and he sent me to see a consultant rheumatologist. This man declared there was nothing wrong with me and implied that it was all in my mind. I felt so apathetic at the time that I didn't protest at his 'diagnosis' and didn't care what he said or thought. I'm a fighter by nature but I was physically and mentally incapable of responding or helping myself. I had reached a point where I couldn't even peel a potato, or hold up my arms to pin up my hair.

After a while I began scouring health books and other health resources for clues and/or answers. The internet was in its infancy then and all I had were library books. Most of the symptoms I had resembled so many other illnesses. It would have been so easy to say 'oh it must be this' or 'yes, it sounds like that'! At the end of the day my condition was 'unidentifiable'. However, through reading these books I learned a lot about the human body and this reading and learning became almost therapeutic because it was so interesting. I learned about the importance of relaxation, a balanced and nutritious diet and vitamin supplements, but, as the months passed, nothing I tried helped in any way. Even the most gentle of exercise exacerbated my symptoms and left me totally weak, exhausted and in severe pain.

By the autumn of that year I had lost my job and was living on benefits. I hated where I lived, became very depressed and just continued to exist in this black hole. In February 1985 my doctor referred me to a different consultant. This consultant took my symptoms much more seriously. He diagnosed me with CFS and added that the condition was a relatively new phenomenon. His last words to me were that my chances of full recovery and getting back into work were minimal. His 'prognosis' had a big effect on me – "never get better". When I came home that day I remembered what other things the consultant had said. "not degenerative and not life-threatening". I realised I had acquired a mystery illness and somewhere deep down inside of me was a vague feeling that I would find my own way to get better, although I didn't have any idea, or inclination, as to how I would even begin to achieve that.

It was Christmas 1986 when I came across an article that described how gentle 'ultra slow' motion stretching exercises could stimulate weak muscles to 'wake up'. An instinctive feeling told me this might be a good precursor to the gentle exercises I had attempted to do before. I devised my own set of ultra slow-motion exercise and did them whilst lying on the floor of my living room every night. After two or three weeks I was able to increase these to twice a day before gradually doing them standing up. After a few weeks of this I began taking short walks outside, building up by a few extra yards each day. A couple of months further down the line I was able to progress to doing very gentle ordinary exercises and by the spring of 1987 my walks had increased to one or two miles, three or four days a week. As long as I took frequent rests on the walks, I was able to complete the goal I had set for that day. There were many days when I did nothing at all, but this, I had discovered, was the key – pacing myself!

My weakness began to improve in very tiny increments, but this gave me hope and encouragement. I never stopped believing that I could get myself better, and every time I remembered the consultant's words 'never get better' it would spur me on in my belief. Progress was slow but positive. However, I was very depressed, had lost every bit of confidence, lost what few friends I had and felt terribly isolated. So when I spotted an advert in the local paper (September 1987), asking for someone to walk a dog for one hour a day, I had a strong feeling that this could be a way to make further progress – the fresh air, the exercise, the companionship of the dog, the sense of purpose and responsibility - and getting away from the black hole that had become my prison. What's more, there would be no pressure from people or employers, I could recover alone. I got the job.

That's how it worked out. Over a period of about six months the one hour walk gradually built up to two hours. I could feel my strength returning. After about nine months it was the whole afternoon, five days a week, much to the delight of the dog owner. As long as I still rested in between and paced myself at home I was able to cope. By this time I was also practicing meditation, which I firmly believe played a major role towards the recovery of my spirit.

It was now Christmas 1987 and the remote possibility of getting back to work had begun to creep into my consciousness. By this time the workplace was changing. I enrolled at the local college to learn some keyboard skills and help rebuild my confidence. It took two years at the college before I was able to feel any competence as I still had to pace myself and my cognitive faculties had suffered immensely. Although recovery was slow but sure, I suffered some major setbacks, mainly emotional, with a very major bereavement thrown in. This added to further years at home, and if it wasn't for these factors I feel I would have made a full recovery much earlier. After many more years at home I returned to college in 1996 and after a further four years of study I gained a teaching qualification. In 2001 I landed a full-time post teaching Information Technology.

I believe that if I had just accepted this illness I would never have got better. However, hindsight tells me that when the body and the mind break down to such an extreme degree then the body has to go through this process. The body in its wisdom takes over. My advice to anyone suffering chronic fatigue is to listen to what the body has said to you and above all, never ever lose the *will* to recover. Life changes will inevitably follow.

Recommended websites
www.kcl.ac.uk/cfs
www.supportme.co.uk

Quote "The way you live and the way you think manifests itself in your body".

Rita Martin

Richard's Story

A structured and logically sound plan for recovery

In his first year of full-time school Richard, aged five, experienced the loss of both his maternal grandparents; and his father had to undergo a triple heart by-pass operation. A gentle, fun loving little boy, he seemed to cope pretty well despite a few troublesome members of his class making life at school difficult at times. He gained good marks but showed signs of being easily distracted from his class work and his concentration did not seem to be too good. At no time was it suggested to us that he had a problem. The troublesome boys in his class began to affect his enjoyment of school and he was never interested in staying on after school for clubs. By 3.30pm he'd had enough and was ready to come home.

He was eight years old when he suffered a severe attack of tonsillitis. He recovered with a course of antibiotics, at the end of which the symptoms, together with a high fever, returned for twenty-four hours. Over the next few months he experienced an increasing amount of time off school with sore throat, tummy ache, nausea, dizziness, severe physical exhaustion and nightmares, which left him sweating and disorientated. He would be fine for about ten to fourteen days, then crash, taking three to four days to recover. He was also emotionally fragile.

With little help from the doctors other than "probably just another virus" we asked for a cytomegolovirus test, as Richard's cousins had both had it and the symptoms seemed similar. The test came back positive for Glandular Fever and the advice given was a dismissive "there's no treatment". I have since learned that the standard test for this, used by GPs, can be unreliable. We decided to reduce his time in school to mornings only to give him a chance to recover.

Richard's condition gradually worsened to the point where he could barely manage two lessons in school for a couple of days a week. I pressed our doctor for a referral to a paediatrician. At this point she appeared to panic and ordered more blood tests, while conceding that Richard might have chronic fatigue syndrome, but repeated her dismissive verdict, "there's no treatment". "But he hasn't been to school for ages" I replied. She just shrugged her shoulders as if to say "so?" Quite coincidentally, it turned out that the paediatrician to whom we were referred, had recently been to a lecture by Dr. David Smith. At this point our luck changed.

A somewhat misleading aspect of Richard's experience of ME was that, in isolation, his physical tolerance was good. By the end of a school holiday he would seem extremely well. At first this led the paediatrician to think that Richard did not have 'full-blown ME' and that we should wait for a while. Looking back (and with the advantage, of course, of hindsight) this was a big mistake. By the time Richard was referred to Dr. Smith, he had been ill for two years.

After our first two hour meeting with Dr. Smith we had no hesitation in entrusting him with Richard's care. By the time the consultation was over, Richard and I were in tears – his from exhaustion, mine from sheer relief that here, at last, was someone who had a credible explanation for this illness and a structured and logically sound plan for recovery.

Dr Smith's understanding and working knowledge of the illness and of what Richard was experiencing was informed and sympathetic. He quickly determined that Richard's cognitive function was more severely affected than his physical function. Richard was referred for assessment by a psychologist to determine the extent of his cognitive function damage. The psychometric analysis revealed that, although he had an IQ on the higher side of average, Richard's cognitive function was affected quite severely. He had a processing deficit, affecting his ability to calculate and follow conversations and storyline; a retrieval deficit, affecting his recall of facts; short term memory deficit and a concentration deficit. It was hardly surprising that he would be physically and emotionally wiped out after two forty-minute lessons.

We began the recovery programme. A small amount of sedating tricyclic anti-depressant was prescribed to help stabilise Richard's sleep. At the same time, sleeping and waking times were regularized, with no napping during the day. Television, the games machine and reading, in excess of his permitted programme periods, were ruled out. His day was broken up into schoolwork periods, physical exercise periods and rest periods. After assessing Richard's activity tolerance level and undercutting it, he began, daily, doing six schoolwork periods of three minutes each and six walking (around the garden) periods of four minutes each – seven days a week. In between activity and rest Richard was allowed to do anything which didn't give rise to symptoms. In his case it was drawing, Lego and listening to talking books.

After establishing this base line for Richard's physical and mental activity (less than he could achieve without making him ill) and introducing regular rest periods during his day, we managed to stabilize his illness. Although this stage can seem extremely tedious, observed faithfully it can soon pay great dividends as the 'crashes' cease and sleep patterns begin to improve. And Richard turned out to be a co-operative patient. This improvement and the knowledge that it was possible to control the illness brought much relief and encouragement to all the family, particularly as Richard's older sister was coping with GCSE and A Levels for the duration of his illness.

A very small dose of prozac was added to his prescription (1ml per day to begin with) as this had been shown to restore brain function, particularly if a patient had been ill for over two years. We then took the programme one step further by very gradually increasing Richard's mental and physical activity, in small increments every three weeks.

During this time we had the services of a Home Tutor from the local Education Authority, who was wonderful. She commented that of all the ME-affected students she had taught, Richard was the only one who was always able to work each day when she came.

We also took our programme out and about on educational visits. On a trip to Hever Castle we did Maths and English in the car, the then ten-minute exercise segment being devoted to getting in and out of the maze. But for Richard, I'd still be in there!

Seven months after he embarked on the programme Richard returned to school for two lessons a day, either side of the lunch break. In our particular case, this was the point at which his recovery slowed down. He began to pick up every virus going around, which knocked him out for longer than a 'well' person. We eventually discovered that this was because he was being subjected to mental and physical bullying by his peer group. We had asked him if he wanted to change schools at the time of his return but he was quite sure he wanted to stay put. We eventually parted company somewhat acrimoniously from his prep school and sent him to a co-educational school. By this time, Richard was attending school full-time but his confidence had taken a hammering.

He took a year to settle into his new school. There were aspects of Year 9, such as a week in the Lake District for which he was quite game, but for which his confidence was not ready and we had grossly underestimated this. The result was shaken confidence and an attack of flu in the Christmas holidays which led to a relapse. Fortunately we very quickly recognized this for what it was and, on Dr. Smith's advice, put him back on the medication for six weeks and after three weeks off school, sent him back mornings only. By Easter he was back full time. Consequently, he repeated Year 9 with some 'provisos', although, even then, I found myself having a set-to with his headmaster, whose attitude was to throw them all in at the deep end and let them sink or swim. I stood my ground and since then Richard has not looked back.

Richard is now twenty-two. He has seven GCSEs, two A-levels and has been in his school's soccer First Team. There is no doubt that due to his illness his academic education has suffered greatly and he missed out on participating in team sports activities at prep school. Looking back now, it is clear that his prep school environment could have been a much more caring one, particularly as far as his peers were concerned, and also a few blinkered staff members. However, in other ways he has gained much. He applied for, against much competition, and was accepted to go on a post-GCSE school humanitarian expedition to Romania. However, before the exams began, he recognized that he had taken on too much and needed a period of tranquility after the exams. He had the courage to acknowledge this and the school organiser was very understanding and released him.

Although we were very sad when he moved out to live in a student house-share while studying for his degree course in Graphic Design, we realised that it was a positive and healthy step to take. Since his recovery, Richard has survived most of life's regular knocks and he shrugs off viruses as efficiently as any other healthy young person.

If I have any advice for other sufferers of ME/CFS it is to keep your life as stress free and as simple as possible. Press your doctors hard for help and don't let them fob you off with lame excuses. Lastly, don't waste your energy being angry that you are ill. Anger and resentment burn up more energy and create more stress than you will ever realise and other angry people just wind you up more. With the right help it is possible for many people to recover. Although prozac is no longer recommended for under sixteen year olds, Richard has suffered no adverse effects whatsoever from taking anti-depressants in the very low doses prescribed.

We could not have achieved Richard's recovery without Dr. Smith's expertise, encouragement and tremendous support. We have had to fight some battles along the way and Dr. Smith has been right behind us every time. Richard may have lost much of his childhood, but Dr. Smith gave him back his life. Dr. Smith has since produced a peer-reviewed paper relating to his treatment of children with ME, which showed an 80.6% recovery rate, believed to be the best result yet published. This can be found in the BMJ publication Archives of Diseases of Childhood October 2003 Vol.88 P894-898.

Most useful aid to recovery - Dr David Smith

Recommended websites
 www.me-cfs-treatment.com
www.me-cfs-recovery.co.uk.
My husband set up these sites for Dr. Smith. It is our way of giving something back and saying "Thank you".

Ann (Richard's mother)

Vicki's Story

Be true to yourself

I feel excited and anxious, a strange combination? The thing is that it actually feels as if I am writing about someone else, that this is a fictional story. It's because I know who I am today and it's *not* the person I used to be , so the truly amazing gift for me is that it's taken my experience of chronic fatigue symptoms to make this transition, to being my true self. I wouldn't change what happened, as my journey has been a revelation to knowing my Self and connecting with my life purpose.

I started to get symptoms of chronic fatigue syndrome when I was seventeen years old. The symptoms were swollen glands and extreme exhaustion, although the doctor found no virus. In retrospect I can see that these symptoms all occurred when I had to do things that I didn't want to do, or when I didn't have the support when life didn't go the way I wanted it to! I can see now that my symptoms were messages from my body telling me that I was not being true to myself in the way I was living my life.

My journey began in a middle-class home in suburban England. I had a normal family but as a highly sensitive person I felt things deeply and wasn't able to express my feelings. I wasn't given the level of emotional security I needed to function successfully in the world, but I am clear today that my family did the best they could at the time and I love them for who they are and know that they had challenging childhoods too. As I got older I lived more and more on adrenaline and I was either in a state of 'flight' (running away and suppressing my emotions) or 'fight' (expressing them in negative and destructive ways). I am clear that I chose my karmic path in order to become the person I am today – a highly sensitive person who lives as authentic a life as I can.

As I continuing to hide my true self, my unconscious started taking action to get my attention. I didn't sleep well; I was crying at night in bed and questioning why I was unhappy and not fitting in with others; I failed my mock A levels; and when Mum was in hospital I took some pills to sleep and cope with the tension - although this was not a suicide attempt but more 'looking for help'. At this time when I got symptoms I used to spend a couple of days in bed and I was fine. Looking back I can see that I wasn't given the skills to cope with stress (how many are?).

I was becoming more and more depressed. It was getting harder to cope and I started to over-eat high-sugar foods secretly, consequently gaining weight, despite being sporty and keeping a good level of fitness. I can see now that it was a way to suppress the fear, anger and anxiety that I felt, and ultimately meant that I had a visible excuse to stay out of normal life and so 'protect' myself.

Looking back,I can see periods of my life when I was acting from my heart and feeling safe, and in those periods I flourished. During the times when I was doing something because 'society said', I felt very insecure and I suffered from symptoms of varying degrees. I hated my university course but didn't know how to ask for what I wanted, always expecting the answer to be 'no'. After my degree, for the first time I asked myself what I wanted and I looked for a career for me, not to 'please' or get attention from others.

I chose to work in book publishing. I believed that business was not going to be an authentic place to be and I wanted to at least be in a business that did something worthwhile. I was still finding it hard to be around people and at work I found my relationships with male authority the biggest struggle. I soon realised that all businesses were the same 'power and control' environments and I was not living my authentic self. I was getting symptoms that were made worse by living in a city as big and impersonal as London. Time off work to recover was never long enough to cause problems and I made sure that my social life was so quiet that I had the energy to work and support myself.

I tried to do normal stuff – I travelled and socialised, but there was always something 'wrong' and I withdrew into myself and my solitary ways. My symptoms didn't come as often if I isolated myself. Any doctor I saw told me I had flu and to rest! I didn't see many doctors as I didn't see the point. Eventually, believing London to be the main cause, I moved to the countryside, but even here I continued to over eat, to stuff down my emotions and continued the year's of yo-yo dieting with a bit of bulimia thrown in. I did have a very loving long-term relationship and during that period the symptoms disappeared. I know now that the love and stability he offered me enabled me to be myself. However, I didn't have the skills and tools needed to maintain such a wonderful relationship.

I knew deep down something was wrong with me, but not how to solve it. So I did what I could and I chose a new career that I believed would fulfil me more than book publishing. I thought working with children would be more 'me' and chose to become a teacher. So I went back to college to become a secondary school teacher. I had a wonderful time for the first five months at college. I was still feeling safe and secure after my relationship and was able to work, rest and play in balance. Then in February my symptoms started to come back during a particularly challenging week of teaching practice. I was crying uncontrollably and most doctors see that as depression, so my doctor offered me Prozac ,which was getting 'trendy' at the time. I left in despair and never actually took the tablets, knowing deep down that it wasn't going to help. I took time out and got back to my 'normal' level of being.

In my first year of teaching, the fatigue and other symptoms worsened. I went to Bristol and the new city and new job were not triggering as many symptoms, so for the first few years I played hockey, made new friends and had a reasonable social life. Then the challenges started to mount and in one year I had some major stuff to deal with. I was made to take a promotion against my wishes, my first serious relationship since London ended and I bought my first flat. I was losing energy quickly and continuing with suppressing my feelings. Depression was a resulting factor again.

Eventually I found the day when I almost couldn't get out of bed. I went to see my local doctor, a wonderful lady. She listened, and for the first time a doctor didn't dismiss me with just flu symptoms, or only depression. She went through the 'diagnosis of exclusion' and I got sick note after sick note as we tried to find a cure for my mystery state. Walking across a road to a supermarket and returning with one bag was all I could manage in my outside life and inside all I could do was feed myself and move from bed to sofa. I chose to make myself get out of bed and extend my movement each day. The doctor was a great support and listened to all my alternative/complementary attempts at healing. I began to read about nutrition, healing, personal development, spirituality, life coaching and so on.

At this time I was totally unable to concentrate, remember facts, or deal with any issues that were not day-to-day survival. I spent from February until September, healing. I went to see a remedial masseur and herbalist. With the massage my body slowly released the tension it had built up. The herbs relieved the tiredness, but I could never see a lifetime of taking herbs as a solution. I also began to meditate and was amazed at the furore going on in my head – it was like a full-scale emergency state in there. Over time my 'over thinking' began to lessen and I was more chilled and less reactive, although I was still waking during the night in anxiety and having nightmares. But I had some tools to deal with the stresses that will always appear in life, relaxing massage and meditation.

I also noticed that certain foods aggravated my fatigue and I began an exclusion diet and saw a kinesiologist to find out what I was allergic to. Armed with a list I began a basic diet of meat, vegetables, rice and potato. Each day I felt stronger and stronger and was able to walk further and further. I also started learning Tai Chi. I progressed slowly and started to feel the energy returning sporadically to my body. Years later I read a great book called 'BodyMind' by Ken Dychtwald which explained how fear in the mind causes tension in the body. I have watched with amazement as over the years my toes have straightened and become mobile, they used to be rigid and curled tightly under. I have found that the catch twenty-two is always that if anything challenges me emotionally, I quickly close down my body, and when my body is closed it is hard to deal with the emotional challenges of life.

Most of this time I have forgotten as they were the darkest hours of my life. I went to see a cognitive behaviour counsellor through the doctor referral service and some of what she said was helpful, although I was still feeling suicidal at the end of our sessions, but not enough apparently to warrant more sessions. I found it easy to cut out sugar and wheat, although at this time there was not the plethora of goods available in the supermarket that there are now. However, Bristol had great health food shops. I lost weight and got stronger as the summer wore on. I was doing affirmations having read Louise Hay's work and other positive thinking books. As the counsellor recommended I started focussing on small steps, I started to decorate my flat. Doing small amounts was challenging but eventually most rooms were repainted and I got better and better.

By September I was determined to return to school teaching and I did. I felt wonderful, energetic, focussed, clear, bright and renewed. My Trade Union had been pretty unsupportive but I returned to virtually a full timetable and head of department responsibilities. My good health lasted about six weeks, and by November I was eating sugar to cope with my symptoms and getting weaker and weaker. Each holiday was major recuperation time again and by

February I was back in bed and on long-term sick leave again. This time I knew that teaching wasn't going to work yet I was uncertain what I could do while I was still getting symptoms. This time the regime of restrictive diet wasn't so easy. The band aid approach worked temporarily but the cause of my condition was not being addressed.

At this time I read about Life Coaching and began training as a coach. It was great as it was virtual learning by conference telephone call and email. I also had my own mentor coach and she, along with the course work, took me through some deep changes which were causing the symptoms. In particular the Coach U Personal Foundation module, which deals with personal boundaries, values, needs, and tolerations, helped me to 'shift'. I was examining who I was and becoming who I really am.

As the thought of how to earn a living and be authentic hung over me, I sold my flat and used the equity to search for my life purpose. I did several workshops, started to train with Brandon Bays, studied Reiki and was attuned to level two, and continued to read. Each day I do self-reiki and clear some of the recent emotions. Eventually I visited Scotland, to experience community life at Findhorn. I stayed doing a three-month creative project and more personal development. I still had low-level depression and fatigue but was maintaining a 'normal' life. I bought a new house and settled down but my life purpose eluded me. I began emotional healing sessions, and was releasing a lot of cellular memories stored from my childhood. A lot of the patterns that would trigger my symptoms are around angry men, authority and feeling responsible. I have spent four years visiting this healer and it has contributed enormously to my holistic healing. It needed to be worked through with action and changes in my everyday life, but the two together propelled me far more quickly to balance and health.

I found one particular spiritual practice that helped me transform my way of thinking completely. I read Don Miguel Ruiz's works and was blown away by how he put into a succinct accessible style exactly what had been happening to me in this lifetime. Miguel explained how we are conditioned by society, parents and teachers to fit into the modern technological world, not as who we are but as who everyone else wants us to be. By doing this we essentially lose ourselves and don't follow our own life purpose but that of pleasing others and fitting in. Miguel gave the Toltec four agreements to use to recover our true self and return to our true being, and so we do not need symptoms any more to tell us we're not being authentic. I found a mentor, Victoria Miller, in USA, and started a virtual apprenticeship. Over the next year and a half I worked the Four Agreements into my way of living and saw tremendous changes and fewer symptoms. I made some of the biggest changes to myself and how I viewed my life. My sense of self love, self trust, self acceptance and self belief grows and grows. This means that I am less likely to put myself into situations that bring up my symptoms. I am more aware of what my authentic self wants and I am more able to respond to my symptoms by making changes.

Mickel Therapy was another piece of my healing puzzle, although very similar to what I had learned in my life coaching. Previously, I was functioning at a normal level for periods of time but eventually I would get symptoms of CFS and need to take time out to recover. It gave me enormous clarity about all I had learned regarding the mind-body connection. I finally understood how my thoughts created my physical body's reactions, yet there were still times when I did all the Mickel Therapy steps and still had symptoms. I eventually realised that I had drifted away from the physical element of my healing. I was not doing Tai Chi and rarely had any massage or body work.

Recently I started doing yoga again and found the breathing and relaxation elements an essential part of my healing. I realised that I literally stop breathing when I am emotionally challenged! To ensure I can function when any challenges come up in life I use either Mickel therapy/life coaching steps to meet my needs or set boundaries, or the body work using breathing and deep relaxation techniques. Ensuring I am relaxed and connecting to my feelings and using them to guide me in the actions I take each day is essential to avoid symptoms. I am a life coach specialising in health, healing CFS and emotional overeating, a spiritual teacher and yoga therapist. I am happy as I explore the paths of life. But whatever choices I make in my life, the only things that matter are that I am authentic, that I am aware of who I am, and I know that if I'm not aware, my symptoms will soon tell me. I also accept that sometimes 'life is a bitch' but it's my choice whether I laugh or cry.

I believe that the holistic approach (mind, body, spirit and emotions) which includes nutrition, exercise, relaxation methods, life coaching and so on, is necessary to heal yourself; and that living a healthy lifestyle includes 80% of what's good for you and 20% of what's not! I also think that healing is a choice, and the path to take is not always the easiest, but it is worth the pain to get to the pleasure. Healing chronic fatigue doesn't come without deep inner work and it's mostly with your own demons.

So some days it's all about breathing practices with yoga postures and other days its about looking at my emotional patterns/beliefs and what I need to change. I think I am an extreme example of this condition. However, the world is not a safe place for anyone and so stress is forever present. Getting the tools to deal with it is essential. I am so glad I've got them and I offer this story so it won't take you quite so long to get the tools too. It's not 'look at me, I'm so happy' – it's about look at me, I am in touch with my feelings, even when I'm feeling sad or angry. Make the choice to become yourself and you will get symptoms to tell you when you're not! I believe we all have our own journey to travel and there are many paths to follow. What I have recounted is my own personal one.

Keep breathing and being true to your self.

Recommended books
"The Four Agreements" by Don Miguel Ruiz
"The Highly Sensitive Person" by Elaine Aron
"The Breathing Book" by Donna Farhi

Recommended websites
 www.miguelruiz.com
www.barbarabrennan.com
www.donnafarhi.nz
www.coachinc.com
www.findhorn.org

Vicki Cook

Marianne's Story

Walking the Labyrinth

When I was first diagnosed with cytomegalovirus and then with ME in early 1990, my GP was very sympathetic. However he was unable to offer me any practical help or prospect of recovery, so I had to look elsewhere. I turned to naturopathic medicine, which works on the principle that your immune system has the innate capacity to heal your body, provided that you help it to do its job. It's a different medical paradigm. I learned that stress of different kinds undermined my health and so I discovered ways to give my body a better chance of recovery.

These are strategies that I used - drinking lots of water, ideally bottled - a body overloaded with toxins needs to use its own transport system to clear them. Clarifying and avoiding foods which I was intolerant to - these included wheat, yeast, cheese, meat, caffeine and additives. Wearing a Bioflow magnet, which seemed to help in detoxification of my body and which even now I find helpful and wear every day. Removing the sources of all chemicals in the home which were causing me problems, such as household cleaning products and bathroom products. I started using safe products by Neways instead. Creating a more energising environment in the home - this I achieved by using plants to improve air quality, especially around major electrical appliances, and keeping the house fairly free of clutter. I also used essential oils in the bath and relaxing music to nurture myself. Discovering ways of living with the illness to the point that it eventually ceased to be a big deal; working with my body and mind rather than battling against the illness. Protecting my body from electromagnetic stress and so reducing fatigue - in 2002 I could not work at a computer for more than fifteen minutes without falling asleep or getting a severe headache; watching television also sent me to sleep. (When in March 2004, I started wearing a Bioguard pendant, a product which apparently protects my body's own electromagnetic pulse from other powerful radiations, I found that I could use a computer without a reaction for hours).

Tapping into many sources of energy - I learned that unlike cars relying on fuel stops, we can obtain energy from sources other than food. Energy comes, for example, from being with people who are good company, from doing things which make us happy, from having a sense of purpose, from spending time enjoying the natural world and from healthy sleep and a tranquil mind. Breathing exercises, meditation and affirmations built up my capacity for dealing with stress and recovered my sense of purpose.

My own process of healing took a long time. Throughout the recovery process I learned a great deal about, not just about my health, but also about my purpose in the world. The healing worked on all levels. My body ached less and worked better and I became less tired. My mind became clearer and more reliable and I found more things to be happy about. The attitude shifts supported and corroborated the healing as it progressed. I came to think of my journey as being like walking a labyrinth. Most people probably think of a labyrinth as a type of maze, but while a maze is designed to confuse and frustrate, a labyrinth is an ancient spiritual tool designed to enlighten. So although I was going around in circles, each circle took me a little closer to my goal, the centre, my healing. Sometimes I seemed to move far away, such as when I had major setbacks. However, as I negotiated the labyrinth, I always kept my goal in mind, if not in sight.

Initially I wanted and expected to find healing that would restore me to the energy levels and quality of life I had enjoyed in my mid-thirties when the ME first struck. I had been teaching full-time, bringing up two young children and looking after a large garden and many animals on our small-holding. In reality, by the time I arrived at a point where being healed was a concept I could even imagine, fourteen years had passed, but my role as a mother had significantly changed and my priorities had shifted. Somewhere along the way, the ME had become not my jailer but my ally. I could choose what I wanted to do. I could combine teaching and writing and still have the time and energy for other things that make me happy, like gardening, walking, cycling, keeping chickens and designing embroidery. I have achieved a quality of life that was not possible before I became ill.

In 1990 I could not walk the length of my garden. Now I am working again. I combine part–time teaching with running a business that promotes health and the environment. I give home tutoring to students who are unable to go to school for health reasons and I do some Primary School supply teaching. In our very exciting business, we provide magnotherapy products to help both people and animals, and a range of products which literally save the environment, either by saving fuel, reducing emissions, or replacing harmful chemicals in the home with those that are safe.

I do my own housework and enjoy cooking and baking for my family. I am also able to maintain a very large garden and grow lots of vegetables. We keep a flock of White Sussex chickens and have just completed our fourth hatch this year. I sing regularly in our parish choir, and attend rehearsals after a day's teaching. We enjoy walking and cycling holidays. I have walked sections of The Ridgeway, the Cornish Coastal Path and our local Greensand Way, as well as shorter walks on other ancient paths. We are planning a cycling holiday in Norfolk this summer using our newly acquired tandem. My husband cycles fifty miles in a day to my thirty miles and this will create a better balance between us!

I always have a pile of books that I am reading, including a course that I am following, and I feel that I am on a steep, but exciting, learning curve. I now have a vision of fitness and purpose which I could not have conceived of without the experience of its opposite; the debility, incapacity, pain and depression of ME.

Anyone, with any chronic illness such as ME, could use the strategies I have used to improve their health. They are generally practical, common sense things, or ancient healing practices. Using all the strategies consistently over time has restored my health completely, and could, I believe, do exactly the same for others.

Recommended websites - www.ecoflow.com

Marianne Oliver

Anna's Story

An upstream paddle against all odds

New! May 15ᵗʰ 2006, Issue 163

"At eight years old I took part in a week long canoeing course at our local club in my home town of Shepperton, Surrey. I loved it. I've always been a very sporty, competitive person. I loved being outside and I get a buzz from training and competing."

Observer Sport Monthly, April 2006 No 74

"… based at the Elmbridge Canoe Club near Weybridge, she won her first European Championship in the K1 marathon in 1997. Her first world championship in that event came in 1999 when she became the youngest woman to win the title. She competed at the Sydney Olympic Games in 2000. In 2001 she won both the K1 (singles) and K2 (doubles) world marathon titles, becoming only the second person in the history of the sport to do that…

She has won a total of seven European and world gold medals. She graduated from Royal Holloway College, University of London with a BSC honours degree in Economics and Management.

…and now living in Walton on Thames she has developed an additional career as a motivational speaker".

When you finished reading those extracts from features in OSM and New! magazine, you may have thought, "what a successful person – isn't she lucky to have all that talent, determination, passion and fame". Well you'd be wrong! My life isn't all passion, perfection and world class achievement - because in April 2003 the whole thing came crashing down around me.

Have you ever woken up when you don't feel ready to start the day? Have you ever felt that you haven't had enough sleep? The energy is there but you just don't feel like activating it? (Monday mornings?) Well, what if it was *worse* than not feeling like getting up? What if you simply *couldn't?* The energy that you needed to roll off the bed, get your feet onto the floor and sitting up, simply wasn't there? Your body was effectively on strike? Imagine if you put your hands on your head - you could easily keep them there for ten seconds, right? What about holding them there for ten minutes? You could probably do that too – they'd get a bit achy and feel tired by the end, but you could do it. But what if you were told to keep them there for ten hours? You probably couldn't, but if you could, they wouldn't just be tired at the end, they would be chronically fatigued. And that is where I was three and a half years ago – I had chronic fatigue syndrome. If you know anything about it, you know someone with it, or you've had it, you'll know that this is serious; it's not an illness that a couple of days in bed is going to cure. This had me out of my sport for *two years!*

I wasn't bad enough to lie in bed, but equally I didn't feel well enough to be out and about in normal every day life. It was like being locked in a half way world, not fully in the 'sick' world but not fully in the 'well' world either. Occasionally I was able to energize myself to do things in the outside world, but would feel thoroughly whacked out afterwards.

The symptoms vary from person to person, but for me included feeling permanently exhausted. It was an effort to do anything. I felt fatigued after very light exercise. I went from racing two and a half hour marathons in a kayak to not being able to do twenty minutes of light paddling in my kayak – the equivalent of a brisk walk. The muscles in my body ached to the degree where it became painful. In fact my muscles ached so much that I couldn't hold my arms up to wash my hair - and we weren't talking for ten hours or ten minutes - more like thirty seconds. Midway I would have to stop and rest. I was a world champion canoeist and it was a chore to wash my hair!

In the beginning I slept loads, often for thirteen to fourteen hours a night. I can recall an occasion when I fell asleep at the dinner table. During another period I suffered insomnia. It was a dismal position – there I was, going from being someone who makes their living from being a professional athlete, someone at the pinnacle of sporting excellence, to a condition that wouldn't allow me to even move on some days. Bit of a bummer being a professional athlete and not being able to move.

And those were just the physical symptoms; the emotional battle was something else.

I'm normally a joyous person and I love life, but this would drain the happiness from me; my stripes would disappear and I would be left with just tears. It really was desperate and if you've had a desperate situation of your own you'll know that two years is a long time and for me it was two years too long.

Initially doctors thought that I had just over-trained, which of course was the most obvious assumption – 'athlete complaining of tiredness and achy muscles'. When you train fourteen to eighteen hours a week this isn't unusual. But this didn't feel like normal tiredness from training. This was fatigue and I knew my training had been quite light prior to this episode of fatigue. I knew in my heart that it wasn't over-training; it felt like something more profound than that, but quite what exactly I didn't know, and neither, it turned out, did many professionals in the industry.

In September 2003 I was eventually diagnosed with CFS. There is a lot of mystery and mystique regarding what it is and its causes. That in itself was one of the most challenging parts of it. How do you explain such intangible things as pain and fatigue? Because I wasn't suffering from cancer or a broken arm people couldn't see or understand it.

Sometimes I wished my skin was see-through so that people could see my pain. I know that people looked at me and thought that I looked perfectly healthy and they wondered what the fuss was about. Some people would even give me a look or a pass a comment like, "it's all in her head", "she's scared", "she's being lazy" or "she really needs to get her act together". Those comments were painful – it was like turning the knife in a wound; for many years I had prided myself in being diligent and industrious and I was the least lazy person I knew! And for those people who thought I was too scared to race, that was crazy - I spent my life living and breathing canoeing.

I put everything on the line for my sport. I had dreamed about winning world titles and Olympic gold medals ever since I was a child. It's pretty hard when everyone is doubting you. But it wasn't really anything new to me; I had always had people tell me I was too small to be a good canoeist, that I would never be big enough or strong enough. My mum would tell me that there was nothing I could do about my size and body shape so there was no point worrying about it. Today I still remind myself all the time, "don't worry about things you can't change. Put your energy into the things that you can change". I realised that I needed to do just the same in this situation. I remember thinking, "that's fine, you keep saying those things because every little comment you make, every little look you give me and every little nudge you give each other is fuel that I'm going to store in my head and use in my darkest days to burn when my symptoms are at their worst. In fact those comments were helping me get better! They gave me more determination to get back to racing and prove them wrong.

Of course I did get back to racing eventually, but it took a long time. Because the general opinion of doctors is that there is 'no cure' I was scared, really scared that I would be trapped by it forever. One doctor, a lady who practised on Harley Street said to me, "Anna, I really think that it's time you listened to your body and accept what it's telling you. Your body has just had enough. You've been pounding up and down the river Thames for too many years and it's just had enough. Your body is finished. Perhaps you should just give up on your sport......that's it, that's the solution - you need to retire Anna, its time to retire. Hang up your paddles." Who was she to tell me it was time to retire? Give up on the sport that I *love*, that I have *dedicated my life to*? I don't think so! That went straight in one ear and out the other.

Of course the doctor wasn't the only one who talked about retiring. Many people who hadn't seen me on the racing circuit just assumed that I had retired. Numerous people asked me if I ever thought about stopping. But not once did I ever think about quitting. Of course I was afraid that I wouldn't be able to return to the sport at the highest level, but at the same time I never gave up hope, it was always in the back of my mind. In fact it's what I used to inspire me and keep my spirits up on my worst days. I'd be having a terrible day, the symptoms would be really fierce, and I'd be getting no respite, wondering when the light at the end of the tunnel was going to appear. I'd be lying on my bed crying and just as I would be ready to give up, the thought of racing again would come to mind and I'd think, "come on Anna, don't give up, don't give up hope, don't give in to this, what about racing? It's your everything, your dream. You can cope with so much more than this."

I used to start picturing myself back on the water, competing at the world championships again. I'd visualise a racecourse, see myself on the start line, picture my rivals and then I'd see the race unfold. I'd see everything. I'd imagine the weather, but I wouldn't just see it, I'd feel it too. I would feel the rain on my skin and feel the wind in my face. And of course I'd always win! I'd imagine that sense of achievement, the sense of fulfilment, the satisfaction in proving all my doubters wrong. The scene would always end with me on the top of the rostrum, with a gold medal round my neck, singing very badly and out of tune to the national anthem! I'd open my eyes at the end and they would have dried up. I'd be smiling and ready to get going again. It was very powerful; not only did it inspire me and cheer me up but also I was creating movies in my mind that I would use when I was racing again.

It was very frustrating that there's so much mystery and mystique about what CFS is. Most doctors said that there was nothing I could do about it except rest. I asked how long I needed to rest for, how long it would go on for? They didn't know the answer, I was just told to rest until it got better. I realise now that it was that lack of knowledge that promoted the fear in me. When you have the knowledge it helps dispel the fear. I didn't have enough information or knowledge about the illness and I was scared. I refused to accept what I was being told. I'd heard stories of people suffering with CFS for ten or fifteen years and I *promised* myself I wouldn't let that happen. *I had to find a way out.* It wasn't in my nature to sit back and just wait – I had to be proactive, I needed to do something about it for my own piece of mind - to know that I was doing everything that I could to find a way out of this miserable condition.

And I guess the key here is that I *believed* that there had to be a way out. I once read a great quote by Norman Vincent Peale who said, "become a possibilitarian. No matter how dark things seem to be or actually are, raise your sights and see possibilities – always see them for they are always there." That reminded me to never lose sight that I would come out of it. Because if the results are down and you lose hope, then you've lost everything.

So I went on a quest to find a solution. I'd been down the conventional route; I'd been to medical experts at the British Olympic Association, to physicians on Harley street. I'd done countless blood tests and consequently had more needles stuck in me than a heroin addict. So with conventional medicine not working, what do you think I tried next? Alternative therapies. You may be sceptical about alternative therapies and I was too, but when you've been to the top of the tree and you want to get back up there, you are desperate and when you're in a desperate situation, you turn to desperate measures.

I started with acupuncture – I had needles in my ears, in my bum and in my toes. I had more needles in me than a hedgehog. In fact I was scared to have a bath in case I leaked! Then I tried yoga – someone suggested that I needed to chill out, go into my body and mind. So I put my legs behind my ears, stood on my head and created a perfect tree pose ready to rival Madonna. I tried crystal therapy and spiritual healing. I saw a number of nutritionists, went on a million different diets and took so many pills I used to rattle. I did homeopathy, more pills. I saw a psychotherapist. And the list went on.

At one stage I saw a nutritionist who said, "Anna you're avoiding all the wrong foods, you're eating all the right foods, you're taking all the supplements I would suggest. You've also done all the tests that I would normally advise. I don't know what else to suggest. Sorry."

My mum, otherwise known as Dr Nela among her friends, usually has a solution to most ailments but she had consulted her 'Guru' book, exhausted the Internet and was still bereft of ideas. Finally I came to the conclusion that I was searching for a needle in a haystack that probably wasn't even there. I was at rock bottom.

One friend called me and said, "Anna, I've been thinking about your illness and I've found the solution. You need to go out, get drunk, get stoned and get laid! Absolute guarantee, works for me every time!" (Of course that was a male friend who had ulterior motives – and sadly it didn't work!).

So I experienced fifteen months of terror and error. What was the solution? Reverse Therapy. I went to Chicago with my sponsors Pindar (an international print and electronic media company based in Scarborough, Yorkshire) for a sports marketing meeting. One of my hosts for the trip was an employee called Jacqueline Kandal. Instantly I connected with Jacqueline who is a wonderful, caring and vivacious lady. I talked to her about CFS and she told me about a friend of hers in the UK who had suffered from ME for a number of years and was currently trying Reverse Therapy.

Just before I left Chicago, Jacqueline handed me some information about the treatment and insisted that I read it and try it. On the long plane journey home I read what Jacqueline had given me and I knew instantly that this was what I had been looking for. No sooner had I got off the plane than I was on the phone booking my first appointment. Thanks to Jacqueline my life was about to change…

Reverse therapy is a relatively new way of addressing the condition. It seeks to find the cause of the problem and not just treat the symptoms. It was discovered that sufferers of CFS, ME and Fibromyalgia are thought to have a disorder in the hypothalamus and adrenal glands. The hypothalamus is a 'master controller' in the brain that controls all bodily functions, from the immune system to the nervous system, as well as the hormones, glands and circadian rhythms. Both the hypothalamus and the adrenal glands in patients of CFS become overactive and when they overwork the muscles, gut, circulation and the immune system, this creates the symptoms that are a part of this miserable condition. There are a variety of triggers that can cause it to overact and they are different for every person. Reverse therapy seeks to stop the hypothalamus from overacting by finding out what the triggers have been.

John Eaton is the Founder of Reverse Therapy UK and I was lucky to work with him directly. Initially I had a reverse therapy session every fortnight and in between sessions I was required to write a daily journal. In the journal I logged all of my activities, my thoughts and feelings, as well as the severity of the symptoms and when they were or were not present. This helped Dr Eaton identify any patterns that were evident and any triggers that might be causing my symptoms. Paradoxically my greatest strengths - being industrious, committed, single minded, focused and dedicated – all of those attributes which helped me become a world champion in the first place - were some of the largest contributors to the demise of my health. I became too consumed with my sport and took this attitude to the extreme. One of my triggers was the fact that I put too much on myself. For example, I was constantly saying to myself, "I have to go training, I have to have the right diet, I mustn't eat this, I mustn't eat that, I must go to bed early…." The list continued and I rarely gave myself a break and on the occasions when I stayed out late or had a few too many glasses of wine I would recriminate afterwards. I had lost the balance and perspective in my life. I spent a large proportion of time training alone, despite the fact that I am a gregarious person and thrive in a social environment.

I lost the very essence of why I started canoeing and competing in the first place – because it is *fun*, because I *enjoyed* it.

Another attribute that I used to credit myself with was vigilance. Hard work for me doesn't just mean training hard six days a week, there is so much more to it than that. Every athlete trains hard, so you continually ask yourself, "am I doing everything that I can? What can I do differently this year that will make a difference? Is this really the path to my desired outcome? Am I getting the right diet, the optimum recovery, have I worked enough on mental preparation, have I really left no stone unturned?" But it's wasn't just once a year that I asked these questions, it was all the time. I was continuously fine-tuning the engine, constantly checking and rechecking. Eternal vigilance, I believed, was the price of success. I was successful and I was vigilant, or at least I thought I was.

The reality however was that I was ignoring some seriously bright flashing lights. There were alarm bells going off all over the place. My body was crying out for me to get a bit of balance in my life, to chill out, to see my friends more, to go out and to let go of some of the conditions. But I didn't listen, I was too consumed by what I was doing and so my body's way of speaking even louder was to give me the symptoms.

Reverse therapy recognises that the mind and the body are connected and that emotional health is linked to physical health. This is evident in that a common trigger for many people is non-expression of emotion. This was true for me. I wasn't good at speaking up and asking for help. Instead I tended to struggle along on my own. Only once in that first year of the illness did I break down and cry in front of someone else. I cried plenty of times on my own, but only once in someone else's company, despite the fact that I have good relationships with my mum, my sister and many close friends. That might seem strange but I think it may be a scenario that many people find themselves in. For example, in business, people regularly take on more and more work – either too much work or tasks which they don't know how to achieve; but they don't ask for help, they keep going on their own without speaking up. In the end they are unable to deliver, they end up blaming other people and when it continues they become more and more stressed until it becomes so big and burdensome that it leads to breakdown. You might wonder why we do this – perhaps it's a fear of showing weakness, looking vulnerable, in a work environment not wanting to look incompetent or un-knowledgeable - for pride? I look back now and realise that I didn't want to let down my guard, to show a weakness or vulnerability. I felt compelled to maintain my athlete poker face, even when deep inside I was desperate for people to see what was behind the mask.

The first winter of my illness I spent two months in Florida, since that is where my coach was based and where I used to do my winter training. Although I wasn't training (I was on a recovery programme set for me by the Olympic team doctor) I was there with my sister Zara, who was training. I recall one day when the symptoms were particularly agonizing. I had the feeling that I was trapped by the illness, suffocating inside my own body. I was morose and melancholic, I cried all morning. Then when I heard Zara return from training I quickly dried my eyes, hoped that she wouldn't notice the redness and when she walked into the room and asked how I was I smiled and replied, "I'm great thanks, how was training?" It was ludicrous, Zara and I are really close, she's my best friend! I realise now that it was just too painful to admit how bad it was, how difficult I was finding it, or worse still admit that I wasn't really coping. As well as that, I didn't want to sound like I was moaning or whinging. I'm usually the one who oozes positivity, the one who feels drained by negativity. I didn't want to drain other people and burden them with my misery and frustration. Then ironically, when I realised I really did need to speak to someone, I found it difficult to find the words to describe the enormity of what I was feeling. Besides, how do I explain to someone else something that I don't understand myself? All of the time however, by not opening up and sharing it with the people closest to me I was just making it worse – I was isolating myself further by not letting people help me.

There were times when I could have wept and should have wept. There were times when I should have said to my coach "this is not good enough" and I didn't. There were times when I could have screamed and shouted and should have screamed and shouted! I didn't have an outlet for my emotions, I didn't open up to my mum or my sister, I didn't ask for or get emotional support from my coach, I wasn't in a relationship at the time, I didn't confide in my friends, I didn't take the help my support team were offering. Despite being surrounded by great people I felt lonely, I was consumed by my sport and there was no balance in my life. There was no outlet for my emotions and no safety valve, so eventually my hypothalamus started working over time and my body just shut down.

What was I to do? There was a mind-body-environment imbalance, which meant I needed to make changes in my life; within myself, in my relationships, in my environment and my work place. I had to make changes because "if you do what you've always done, you'll get what you always got". And I'd had enough of what I was getting! I started to realise what I was doing through the journal and Dr Eaton. When I had the courage to open up to people, show some vulnerability and allow those people who desperately wanted to help, to help me, I started to get better. The best bit was opening up to people, sharing it with them and letting them help me. It was liberating. And even better than that, they didn't judge me. They didn't think that I was weak or that I was a lesser person because I was scared and I cried; they were just very supportive.

I started reverse therapy in September 2004 and I have to admit that it wasn't easy. It took me a while to fully comprehend what it was about and how it worked. Also the sessions in the beginning were emotionally draining and painful (not physically). This was because Dr Eaton was incredibly intuitive, he was precise and he challenged my core and the habits that I had developed over years. I had to work hard at the changes that needed to be made and I wasn't always successful at first. Fearing the symptoms creates a vicious circle and eliminating this fear was one of the biggest challenges. However, with the help of my family, friends and sponsors Pindar, who stood by me throughout the illness and covered all of my medical bills, I persevered and by Christmas my symptoms were fairly mild.

In January I started light exercise (fifteen to twenty minute run or paddle in my kayak). By March I was training moderately (low intensity training, forty-five to sixty minutes once a day, five days a week) and although I still had some mild symptoms at this time, the difference was like night and day.

I built up my training slowly and went from strength to strength. The more I trained the more my confidence grew and the more my fear of the symptoms diminished. Within ten months of starting reverse therapy I had already recaptured my status as British number one and re-claimed my European title.

On the 23rd of July 2005 I became European champion again for the third time. It was incredible. It had been a remarkably rapid turnaround and I had to pinch myself to check that it was real. Immediately after the race when I hugged Zara and she attempted to explain the tears that were pouring from her eyes, she said, "this one meant so much more (than the other European titles)." She wasn't wrong.

Although I had defeated chronic fatigue syndrome and I had National and European titles under my belt, the battle wasn't over, there was still a world title waiting to be claimed.....

On the 1st of October after another two months of training I was finally on my way to Australia for the 2005 marathon racing world championships. This is what I came back for; to win world championships and gold medals. On the darkest most desperate days of my illness this is what I focused on – world titles. Just when I thought there was no more light at the end of the tunnel, when I was ready to give up, I focused on what inspired me – being the best in the world.

The day before the race I had a moment of reflection. I recalled a time just thirteen months before when I was still scared that I would never compete in a world championships again. Yet there I was, just seven and a half months after recommencing training and I was about to compete at the World Championships, going into the race as the British number one, the European Champion and the favourite for the World Championships. It was an enormous achievement just to be there and I reminded myself that whatever happened the next day, it had been a fantastic year already. I went to bed that night feeling nervous but excited.

I woke up on race day with butterflies in my stomach. I really didn't feel like putting any food in my stomach, but I had to eat breakfast - I had an eighteen mile race to do! So I forced some down. The race was in the afternoon and about an hour and half before my race I began my warm up. Then about twenty-five minutes before the race, after changing my mind about five times about what kit I was going to wear, going to the toilet fifteen times and checking my boat through forty times, I was finally ready to head to the water. Not that I'm indecisive or paranoid in any way! I headed to the dock. My coach put me on the water, gave me his final words of wisdom and finally I was alone. I had just under twenty minutes to finish my warm up and collect my thoughts. Soon enough we were called to the start line, we lined up in boat number order and before I knew it the gun went: BANG! I got off to a good start and I did enough to make it into the front group.

Within twenty minutes the leading pack had whittled down to just three. I realised that the other two girls were European, (a Pole and a Hungarian), girls I had raced and beaten at the European Championships two months before. It was looking good. All of a sudden I started to get a bit carried away, I was saying to myself, "that's it, the race is mine, it's in the bag". Foolish! I reminded myself not to be so arrogant. Confidence is good, over confidence can be dangerous. I drew my attention to the fact that we had only done about three miles and there were fifteen more to go, a lot could happen. A wise man once said, 'life is a marathon not a sprint.' Very apt.

The race consisted of four laps and four portages, (a portage is where you have to get out of your kayak and run with it for two hundred metres before re-entering the water for the next lap), each lap being 7.2 kilometres long. My major plan for the race was to lead into the final portage, sprint round and make a break. I'm a pretty good runner so it normally works. It was my usual strategy, but for a variety of reasons I hadn't used it at the European Championships, so it had been four years since I had physically put it in to practice. However, I had done it a thousand times in my head. I had created those movies and I'd watched them over and over again. All I needed to do now was press play…

We were about a hundred and fifty metres away from the final portage when I took the lead; I arrived at the portage, leapt out of my boat and totally focused I ran. I was ready to embrace the hardest part of the race. Imagine this, you've already been racing for an hour and three quarters, you get out of the boat and run with it as rapidly as you can for two hundred metres, the first hundred and seventy metres being on grass around a bend and then the last thirty metres on sand.

Just as your legs are getting tired it gets even tougher – the sand completely zaps the energy from your legs. You get back in, your legs have ceased up, your arm is tired from carrying the boat, your lungs are bursting and then you have to pull away and paddle as fast as you can. I managed to establish a one hundred metre lead but I knew that if I relaxed they would catch me. I paddled hard but this was the bit that hurt – the pain was kicking in big time. Then I realised that I'd been there before, in a number of races and in a thousand training sessions. I remembered that this is what I trained for; on all of those days when it was cold and rainy and I didn't really feel like going out training, when I was tired and lacked motivation, this is what I would focus on – being able to push through the pain barrier in the last six kilometres of the world championships, winning world titles, this was the end I had in mind. So I paddled as fast as I could and I went through the pain barrier.

Finally I entered the home straight. There was no chance of anyone catching me now. The challenge was to maintain my focus, because all of a sudden I was distracted by the thought of another world title and that made me emotional. This was not the time to be getting emotional. I hadn't won yet. I blocked it from my mind, but seconds later it came back and then I started thinking about what my victory gesture would be. Can you believe it? I hadn't even crossed the line. I needed to focus. I did and finally after two hours and sixteen minutes of racing I crossed the line in *first place – world title number four*. I threw my arms in the air and gave a yelp of joy and relief.*

I got off the water. My parents, my sister and my auntie were all there with tears in their eyes and me with a lump in my throat. It meant so much to have them there to share the moment with. They had seen me during the doldrums and they knew what this meant. It was all rather overwhelming and it took a while for it all to sink in. When it did, that feeling was like nothing else - words cannot describe it. I just know that it was sweeter than any of the other victories I have ever achieved.

I had climbed the largest and most arduous mountain to achieve that particular gold medal. It wasn't an easy journey, but nothing worth achieving is ever easy. Success, I realise, is to be measured not so much by the position that one has reached in life, as by the obstacles which one has to overcome whilst trying to succeed. So when you are having one of your own dark and desperate days, remember, NEVER give up!

The month after the world championships I went on to win the inaugural Champions Award at the 2005 Sunday Times Sportswoman of the Year Awards. To be recognised in this way was very special and a real honour. It was the ultimate triumph in a year that turned out to be better than anything even I could have dreamed of. I am now in full training for the 2008 Olympic Games in Beijing. The competition will be fierce and the tide against me strong, but I can handle that thanks to training, the right attitude and … I've got the energy!

Dedicated to my parents, my sister Zara, the Munchkins (Cara, Caroline, Laura, Marilyn and Sarah) and Andrew Pindar, without whom this story wouldn't have had the fairy tale ending that it does. Anna would also like to thank SpinVox for supporting her.

*If you would like to see video footage of this last section of the race please go to my website and click on the multimedia link. (See 'More about the authors' at the back of the book).

Most useful aid to recovery - Reverse Therapy

Recommended book - "ME, CFS and Fibromyalgia – The Reverse Therapy Approach" by John Eaton.

Recommended website - www.reverse-therapy.com

Quote - "Don't rush the harvest. If you work with reverse therapy, if you believe in it and embrace it fully, you'll reap the rewards in the end." Andrew Pindar

Anna Hemmings

MORE ABOUT THE
AUTHORS

Foreword

Dr Jacob Teitelbaum is the Medical Director of the National Fibromyalgia and Fatigue Centers, USA. He lectures to patient, physician and research groups internationally. He is the senior author of the landmark studies "Effective Treatment of Chronic Fatigue Syndrome and Fibromyalgia - a placebo-controlled study" and "Effective Treatment of CFS and Fibromyalgia with D-Ribose". He is also author of the best-selling books "From Fatigued to Fantastic!", "Three Steps to Happiness! Healing through Joy" and "Pain Free 1 – 2 – 3 - A Proven Program to Get YOU Pain Free!" (McGraw Hill, 2006) www.vitality101.com   www.fibroandfatigue.com

Stories

Alexandra Barton lives in the UK with her husband and two children. She works as a life coach, counsellor and nutritional therapist helping people with CFS/ME find their own individual route back to health and happiness. Her website is www.alexbarton.co.uk and she can be emailed via her website or contacted on: 0845 051 4658. Alexandra compiled and edited "Recovery from CFS – 50 Personal Stories", which is also available as an ebook on www.cfsrecoverystories.com .

Alex Howard is the Founder and Clinical Director of The Optimum Health Clinic, 1-7 Harley Street, London, W1G 9QD. The Optimum Health Clinic offers a number of free CDs worth of information for people with ME. See website www.FreedomFromME.co.uk. Alex Howard also runs an M.E. Recovery Group where he interviews someone with an inspirational recovery story by conference call every two weeks – more information can be found at www.SecretsToRecovery.com. Alex lives in North London and in addition to working with patients and supporting the clinic team, Alex is deeply passionate about his work running psychology based training courses.

Anna Hemmings is from London, a six time world champion canoeist and motivational speaker. After overcoming CFS she signalled a miraculous return to fitness by regaining her status as the world's leading marathon canoeist at the Marathon Racing World Championships. Anna has gone on to win a hat-trick of three world titles in a row (2005, 2006 and 2007). The latest medal is her sixth gold since 1999 confirming her status as Britain's most successful ever female canoeist. She now has an incredible 11 World and European Championship medals, 9 of them gold. Anna's achievements were recognised at the 2005 Sunday Times Sports Woman of the Year Awards, where she won the Champions Award and again in 2007 when she won the BBC London Sports Personality of the Year Award. Anna would like to thank her family and fiancé Neil for helping her get to where she is today, and her sponsors Pindar and SpinVox for having faith and supporting her. For more information on Anna and her story please go to www.annahemmings.com.

Barbara Rivers is 72 and she works hard in her garden. She loves to walk her dogs and spend time with friends and family. She lives in Cheshire, UK.

Bob Mantz Jr. is a health researcher and interviewer as well as an editor for Curezone.com - the second most visited alternative health site on the internet. He's interviewed doctors, herbalists and alternative health practitioners for web broadcast and CDs. His writings have appeared in numerous newspapers, newsletters and websites. Bob resides in Cranbury and is the President of Princeton HR Consultants, www.princetonhrconsultants.com. He uses herbs from www.return. to/organicherbs and vitamins/supplements from Dr. Christopher via www.superfood.andmuchmore.com. Contact Bob via his website: www.bobmantz.com .

Chris Mole is a freelance web designer and Internet marketer, based in Ashburton, New Zealand. His company, Ace of Webs (www.aceofwebs.com), helps businesses to market themselves more effectively on the Internet. Chris also owns two websites dedicated to CFS and hypoglycemia, at www.chronicfatigue-help.com and www. hypoglycemia-diet.com.

Christine Goodall continues to run a 'parrot boarding house' and is a busy artist and craftswoman living in Bristol, UK. To talk to Christine, or for commissioned artwork, telephone: 0117 950 8059.

Christine Patient very much enjoys having her health back. Her illness and recovery gave her a different direction in life and enabled her to achieve goals which she had previously only been able to dream about, those of learning to swim and learning to play the piano. Christine lives in Essex, UK".

Christine Whiteman lives in Watchett, UK. She is a retired farmer's wife, now aged 65 and feeling as fit as she did at 50. She keeps busy doing voluntary work with the elderly, and makes sure that she watches her diet and doesn't eat too much sugar or yeast. Christine is happy for anyone to contact her. Telephone 01984 640 825

Dr Clare Fleming is a wife, mother, doctor and photographer. She returned to medicine in 2005 after a 15 year career break, during which she enjoyed family life and a range of other activities. She currently works in general practice and alcohol addiction. She has edited two reports from the National Task Force on CFS/ME, and contributed to the Action for ME residential rehabilitation courses for people with CFS/ME. Clare lives in Bristol, UK.

David Jameson lives in a small town in Canada with his wife and dog, running his own business (www.groupboard.com) developing web conferencing and distance learning software. He hasn't had any CFS symptoms for over six years. David is the author of "Mind-Body Health and Stress Tolerance" and has a website: www.mind-body-health.net.

Dr David Mason Brown MB ChB is the Consulting Director of "In-Equilibrium" www.in-equilibrium.co.uk . In-Equilibrium is a Stress Management Consultancy which offers workshops on stress, lifestyle, energy and so on. Dr Mason Brown's website is www.cfs-me.co.uk and he is happy to give telephone consultations for support. Email: drmasonbrown@aol.com For one to one consultations see website: www.medicalternative.com/david_mason)brown.html. .Dr Mason Brown lives in North Berwick, East Lothian, Scotland www.north-berwick.co.uk/index.asp

Diana Daniele is the President of Diana Daniele Communications, a public relations and marketing firm in Los Angeles. She is currently at work on a book of poetry . She lives with her husband, son and new baby in Southern California. She welcomes your feedback at: diana.daniele@roadrunner.com.

Emma lives in Sydney, Australia.

Fiona Agombar teaches yoga full-time and specialises in teaching yoga to people with ME. She runs retreats in England and Turkey and details of these can be found on her website www.fionaagombar.co.uk. Fiona also travels and studies yoga in India. She is the author of the book and CD "Beat Fatigue with Yoga", and lives in London, UK. Email Fiona at: fionaagombar@fionaagombar.co.uk or fagombar@fagombar.co.uk

Helen Long is now a healthy 20 year old. She is studying part time, and working part time in an after school club. She has a full social life and is very involved in Green politics. She hopes to go to university and then find a job relating to politics and the environment. Her mother, **Fran Long,** wrote Helen's recovery story and lives in Kent, UK. Fran has been an NHS nurse for 30 years. The ME experience has made her question the authority of the medical professions, and given her a respect for complementary medicine. She found advice and support from other members of the ME association invaluable, and so welcomes enquiries about any topic raised by this story. She can be contacted on 01732 506096 or flongs@btopenworld.com

Howard is primary carer for his disabled son and full time dad to his very healthy younger brother. Howard is a high school chaplain. He lives with his wife and two boys in Toowoomba, Australia and is more than happy for anyone to make contact with him concerning his journey of freedom from chronic fatigue syndrome. Email: hb4jc@aapt. net.au

Ian is now retired and living in Buckinghamshire, UK. He enjoys country rambles and writing memoirs.

Jessica Crabtree now feels she can take part in any type of activity and is currently developing her singing, dancing and musical skills. She keeps fit by attending three types of dance classes a week, ballet, hip-hop and tap. She plays violin, piano, guitar, saxophone and drums is to be her newest instrumen; most of these instruments she plays to a grade eight and grade six standard. She sings in her school choir and is a member of the ac-up Pella group. She arranged the music and rehearsals for her school house instrumental and house song competitions and hours of work and lots of energy were required for this. She has written and recorded a number of songs, two of which relate to her feelings as an ME suffer. Jessica's life is very busy. She is taking her A2 in music and ceramics in summer 2008, she is a part time boarder and is involved with many activities in school. She also has a job at Tesco one day a week, serving on the tills. She is hoping to continue her studies at Leeds College of Music where she wants to develop her musical skills. Her aim for the future is to be singer songwriter.

Jess Michael is know to many as 'The Raw Lifestyle Coach,' and is a raw food author and managing director of Total Raw Food Ltd, the online natural health superstore. She is the UK's leading raw food promoter and lectures at many UK raw food and vegan festivals, whilst also running her own very popular raw food events. Jess is the author of a range of ebooks including 'Total Raw Food: The Complete Guide For Beginners' and is featured regularly in the media after turning her life around from CFS. As a raw food coach her clients range from CFS sufferers to celebrities, athletes and giant blue chip organisations. Jess is based in Brighton, and lives in her 100% raw vegan home, which she shares with her fiancé and business partner Tom Fenton. Contact Jess via her websites www.totalrawfood.com and www.jessmichael.com.

Joanna Hayes is currently setting up her own business as a Sports Rehabilitator and lives in the East Midlands, UK.

Joy Anthony is now 76 and lives in Jersey. She continues to take Armour Thyroid and adrenal supplements when needed. She loves to spend time with her friends and going shopping. Joy is happy to be contacted. Telephone: 01534 853 012 or email: lafolie2fl@hotmail.co.uk

Karen Hallam lives in Leicestershire, UK, with her husband and two children aged 4 and 7. She has a part time admin job and works three days a week. She is also training in hairdressing and attends college twice a week. Karen is happy to be contacted on her email address: Karen@gleesons-posinst.co.uk .

Katherine Austen is enjoying life running an organic, chemical free Bed and Breakfast in Cornwall. www.davidshouse.co.uk Email: info@davidshouse.co.uk

Telephone 01208 814514 or 07831 514 811

Lilla is currently developing her creative practice in the visual arts and is studying for an M.A. in printmaking and book arts. Since applying the Lightning Process training she's been back to India to work (which was totally knackering in a non-ME way), is going to university for the first time, has just received her bus pass, and says ... rock on! Lilla lives in Bristol, UK

Lizzie Neal graduated from the University of Sheffield this summer with a 1st Class Honours degree in English Language with Linguistics. She is still living in Sheffield while she completes a PGCE in Post Compulsory Education, so she can teach basic literacy and English to adults. By June 2008 she will have her qualified teacher status and has a feeling that she will be heading off to explore the world a bit more – New Zealand is calling.

Louise lives with her husband, daughter (17) and son (11) in Norfolk, UK. Soon after recovery she applied for a new job and works part time in a GP practice. She loves going on family holidays abroad and in her spare time she enjoys meeting up with friends. Feeling well means that keeping busy and having fun is back on the agenda! Louise is happy to be contacted. Email: Milnerlouise@aol.com

Maggie Leathley lives in Sheffield and has been fully recovered for 5 years. She works for a cancer charity training and supervising volunteers. Maggie works part-time because she is also carer to her 18 year old son who has had ME for 5 years. She is looking forward to celebrating her 50th birthday in full health, as opposed to her 40th birthday when she was very ill and spending 22 hours of every day in bed.

Mandy Robson is now 39 and works as a paralegal for a busy debt recovery unit within a leading law firm in Newcastle upon Tyne. She lives in Hedgefield with her partner, seven year old son and a two year old dog which she enjoys walking twice a day for forty minutes - something that would have been unthinkable a few years back!

Margaret is an author and she lives in Suffolk, UK

Marianne Oliver is the author of "Be Free of M.E. – a Healing Journey". This gives a detailed account of her own process of healing and the strategies she applied. In it she reviews a dozen therapies, twenty books, a course and other resources which have been vital to her recovery. Website: www.befreeofme.co.uk Email: marianne@befreeofme.co.uk

Matthew Benton is now working full time in local government IT, with a full time social life and another full time job restoring his Victorian house and another starting a web company. He also exercises and plays sport regularly, but is confident he can do all of this without fear of the CFS returning." Matthew lives in Bristol, UK, and has a website www.beatcfs.info.

Maureen lives in San Francisco, USA

Max Rivers of 'Two Rivers Mediation' is a professional couples mediator who has a private practice focused on helping couples navigate their difficult conversations. He is healthy, recently married and lives in Philadelphia, USA . www.TwoRiversMediation.com

Mike Roger works for a financial firm and lives in New Jersey, USA. He has maintained a low carbohydrate diet and the whole family thrives on it. Sugar and flour are not allowed in the house.

Monique is currently in the process of starting her own design company specialising in bespoke contemporary furniture with a classical twist. She plans to work part-time so that she has time to enjoy her other passions of gardening, cooking and travelling. Monique lives in Holland

Naomi Cooper lives in Gosport, Hants, UK with her husband Martin. She has 2 grown up sons and a daughter in law. She has made a CD of Christian relaxation and meditation exercises. She has a website www.jonc.me.uk/relax through which you will see more of her life story. She can be contacted through that or by email: relax@jonc.me.uk

Norah Bleazard lives in Ontario, Canada www.corelinkwellness.ca

Patricia Franklin lives in Shrewsbury, UK. For copies of her programme "ME and my Fidgets" send your name, address and a cheque for £4 to: Mrs. P. Franklin, 18 Forest Way, Shrewsbury, UK, SY2 5RP.

Paul Wheeler lives with his girlfriend and together they run a market stall business selling sweets and cards etc. He runs three or four times a week and lives in Portsmouth, UK. Paul is happy to be contacted. Email: paulwheeler38238@aol.com

Ri lives in Arizona, USA. When given the opportunity, he helps teach people through nutrition consulting, detoxification, in-home-cooking-lessons and food store walk-abouts as he likes to call them.

Richard is now twenty four and has a degree in Graphic Design. He is sharing a house with four others in Southampton and holding down a job while trying to get established as a freelance illustrator. Having missed so much schooling he has had to grow up at a much faster pace, but has stayed well and survived all the things that life threw at him in his late teens and early twenties. Being the last to leave the nest his mother, Ann, probably worries more about him, but she suspects that is fairly normal. Ann can be contacted through two websites: www.me-cfs-recovery.co.uk and www.me-cfs-treatment.com.

Rita Martin gained her teaching qualifications in the year 2000 and immediately landed a post at her local college where she has spent seven happy years. In 2003 she met a wonderful man and they became great partners. Shortly after getting her teaching job she sought help from a Bowen Technique therapist regarding a frozen shoulder. She had suffered with her shoulder for many years, prior to developing fibromyalgia. This therapy completely resolved the problem, permanently, so she decided to train and qualify in this remarkable therapy and now runs a part-time practice. The Bowen Technique is a very gentle therapy which works on the entire muscular system and related tissue. It is renowned for helping people with fibromyalgia/ME but Rita has never personally treated anyone with this condition. Rita lives in Leeds, West Yorkshire and is happy for anyone to contact her via her website: www.boweninleeds.com.

Rob Fairfield is now back at university studying his Diploma in Architecture. He lives in Oxford and will be a fully qualified architect in three years. Having recovered from ME six years ago, Rob is happy and is enjoying life again. Rob's Mother, Diane (the author of the story), is also happy. She lives in Oxfordshire and is a support teacher at the local primary school. Rob would welcome contact by e-mail to rewfairfield@gmail.com.

Stuart Runham lives in Bedfordshire, UK. He returned to full-time work five years ago as an Aeronautical Engineer. It is the same job he had before he became ill - he had a very understanding employer! The job is mostly desk-based, with a lot of travel. He is married to a very understanding wife who had a difficult time when he was ill, and they would like children in the future. They both enjoy life as much as they can, with holidays in the countryside, walking and the general outdoors. He also enjoys creating computer art and animation and when he has the time, he sits down to read a good book. Contact Stuart on stuart@stu-runham.co.uk website www.stu-runham.co.uk .

Susie Novis is a Life and Happiness Coach, NLP Practitioner and Mickel Therapist living in Yorkshire, UK. To contact Susie at the 'Spirit of Success' telephone 01723 374 190 or email: susie@mickeltherapy.com or spiritofsuccess@btinternet.com. The website www.thespiritofsuccess.co.uk is coming soon. Susie lives in Yorkshire, UK.

Tom Bickley is now 16 and in the sixth form at school studying for his A'levels. He lives in North Warwickshire, UK with his parents and sister and enjoys playing guitar in a band. To contact Tom email: Tom.bickley@mac.com. To contact his mother Kim, who wrote his story, email: r.bickley@virgin.net.

Tracey Cheetham lives in South Yorkshire with her husband Tim. They have three young children. Tracey is a researcher at the university of Huddersfield where she is working towards her PhD. She and her family frequently get very dirty indeed! Tracey is happy to be contacted via email: t.c@lycos.com

Ute Wieczorek-King is a business coach who specialises in time and stress management and work-life balance. She helps people to be more effective in business and get more out of their work/life. She coaches people face-to-face, as well as over the phone, and is based near Windsor, Berkshire, UK. She is happily married with three grown up children and enjoys travelling and learning new things. Her website is www.uwk.biz and she can be contacted on: +44 (0)7729 212299 or via email at ute@uwk.biz.

Vicki Cook is a life coach who specialises in health, healing and self care. She is also a yoga therapist and incorporates body work with coaching to ensure that clients have a holistic toolbox for lifetime health and happiness. She currently lives in Edinburgh, Scotland. Her website is www.golightlycoaching.com.

GLOSSARY

Action for M.E: A UK charitable organisation for people affected by CFS/M.E.

Adrenal Glands: Two glands the size of walnuts which sit on top of the kidneys. Their primary function is to prepare the body for acute and chronic physical and emotional stress. These hormones influence nearly every bodily function.

Adrenaline: A hormone produced by the adrenal glands to facilitate sudden physical activity in emergency. One effect of adrenaline is to raise blood sugar.

Bio-terrain analysis: A simple test or urine, blood or saliva, to give you an overview of the entire internal environment of your body.

Candida Albicans: A yeast like fungi which can get out of control if you have a weakened immune system.

Chronic Fatigue Syndrome: CFS is characterised by a "severe disabling fatigue which lasts for more than six months, made worse by minimal physical or mental exertion, and for which there is no adequate medical explanation". There are also many other symptoms. CFS is sometimes called M.E. (Myalgic encephalomyelitis)

Clonus: Involuntary muscle contractions

Coeliac Disease: A life-long inflammatory disease of the intestinal lining caused by intolerance of the protein gluten, found in wheat, rye and barley.

Dopamine: A brain chemical associated with feelings of motivation

Fasciculations: A small, local, involuntary muscle twitch

General Practitioner (GP): English family doctor

Gluten intolerance: Intolerance of the gluten protein found in wheat, rye and barley

Glycaemic index: A ranking system for carbohydrates based on their effect on blood sugar levels

Gut dysbiosis: An imbalance of bacteria in the digestive tract

Hypothalamus: A region of the brain that regulates homeostasis. It regulates thirst, hunger, water balance, blood pressure, body temperature and links the nervous system to the endocrine system.

Hypoglycaemia: A condition where the level of sugar (glucose) in the blood drops below a certain point. May be difficult to distinguish from neuropsychiatric illness due to symptoms.

Kinesiologist: A therapeutic system of muscle testing to access what is happening in the body

Klebsiella: Klebsiella bacterial infections tend to occur in people with weakened immune systems

Lightning Process: A training programme which combines concepts from neuro-linguistic programming, hypnotherapy, life coaching and osteopathy to allow you to address any area of your life where you experience being stuck, or would like to be more successful.

M.E. Association: A UK charitable organisation for people affected by CFS/M.E.

Mickel Therapy: A specialised approach to health which requires no medication, supplements, dietary change or hands-on modalities. It is not hypnotherapy or psychotherapy but an individual approach addressing wellness and the prevention of illness.

Myalgic Encephalomyelitis: M.E. is characterised by "severe disabling fatigue which lasts for more than six months, made worse by minimal physical or mental exertion, and for which there is no adequate medical explanation". There are also many other symptoms. M.E. is sometimes called CFS (chronic fatigue syndrome).

Orthomolecular medicine: A practise of preventing and treating disease by providing the body with optimal amounts of substances which are natural to the body.

Prolactin: A hormone produced by the pituitary gland

Reflexology: A complimentary therapy working on the feet to help heal the whole person

Reverse Therapy: An educational process which teaches people how to eliminate symptoms by understanding and acting on the 'message of the symptom' - what Bodymind is trying to 'say' through the symptoms in order to warn, guide and protect the individual.

Rolfing – A method of hands-on tissue manipulation and movement education.

Serotonin: A brain chemical associated with feeling happy and calm

Shop Mobility: A UK charity allowing you to borrow wheelchairs and disabled scooters

INDEX

(Therapies mentioned in the stories)

Absorbing interests: 205,
Acceptance: 84, 244, 307,
Acupuncture: 22, 27, 58, 76, 111, 151, 190, 256, 258, 259, 276, 277, 278, 319,
Adrenal glands: 65, 66, 69, 70, 94, 234, 287, 321,
Adrenal hormones: 73
Adrenals: 65, 66, 69, 73,
Adrenaline: 4, 10, 12, 13, 15, 16, 52, 65, 66, 89, 128, 302
Affirmations: 305, 272, 311,
Alpha state: 98, 100
Amalgam fillings: 170, 250,
Amitriptyline: 62, 96, 131, 133, 228,
Anti-candida diet: 64, 119, 220, 275
Anti-depressants: 103, 105, 106, 209, 210, 213, 219, 299,
Anti-fungals: 185,
Antibiotics: 51, 100, 109, 185, 246, 271, 278, 295,
Apple Cider Vinegar: 114
Artenox D: 234
Artenox M: 234
Autogenics: 63, 98
Ayurvedic medicine: 179, 184,
Balanced diet: 181
BE Kit: 138
Belief: 76, 97, 100, 274, 293, 307, 308
Bio-terrain analysis: 56
Blood Group Diet: 186, 233,

Bowen Technique: 279, 339
Breathing exercises: 133, 311
Carbohydrates: 11, 60, 64, 65, 66, 67, 68, 180, 181, 182, 248, 249, 338
Cayenne: 114, 116
Chemical free diet: 282, 283
Chinese herbal medicine: 171, 190, 258, 259,
Chlorella: 54
Christian faith: 210, 279, 280, 338
Co-enzyme Q10
Cod Liver Oil: 121
Cognitive Therapy: 97, 99
Colonic irrigation: 63
Core Stability ball: 277
Cortef: 113,
Cortisone: 113, 114
Counselling: 63, 151, 186, 210, 269
Cranial osteopathy: 190
Crystal healing: 151,
Curezone: 114, 116, 332
Dairy-free diet: 236, 241
DHEA: 111
Diet: 11, 12, 13, 21, 22, 35, 36, 51, 54, 56, 58, 60, 61, 63, 64, 65, 66, 67, 68, 69, 70, 76, 82, 99, 103, 105, 106, 107, 108, 111, 113, 115, 119, 121, 152, 158, 173, 175, 178, 179, 180, 181, 182, 183, 184, 186, 199, 205, 207, 208, 214, 219, 220, 227, 231, 233, 234, 236, 237, 238, 240, 241, 248, 249, 253, 255, 256, 261, 262, 269, 273, 274, 275, 277, 278, 281, 282, 283, 285, 291, 303, 305, 306, 320, 321, 322, 333, 338, 343,
Echinacea: 274
Efamol: 209, 210
Emotional Freedom Techniques: 151
Enada NADH: 52
Energy medicine: 101
ENT surgery: 271
Essential Fatty Acids: 233, 234, 249
Exercise: 2, 7, 58, 63, 85, 92, 99, 107, 112, 113, 116, 128, 133, 141, 173, 183, 188, 191, 192, 193, 205, 213, 314, 237, 239, 243, 244, 259, 261, 262, 277, 280, 285, 292, 293, 297, 298, 308, 311, 315, 325, 337, 338
Faith: 146, 149, 178, 184, 209, 210, 279, 280,
Fats: 12, 13, 61, 64, 65, 66, 67, 68, 69, 99, 180, 181, 182, 185, 199, 233, 234, 249,
Fidget exercises: 133, 137, 338

Selenium: 185, 234
Shop Mobility: 343, 6
Snake venom: 206
Spirituality: 63, 163, 202, 210, 214, 217, 218, 271, 304, 306, 308, 320,
SSRIs: 7
Supplements: 46, 52, 54, 55, 56, 58, 60, 61, 63, 64, 73, 76, 111, 151, 152,
170, 171, 172, 199, 209, 210, 220, 227, 233, 238, 249, 274, 276, 279,
291, 320, 333, 336
Swimming: 28, 152, 277,
T3: 72, 73, 113, 114
Tai Chi: 144, 305, 307
Thyroid hormones: 63,
Thyroxine: 66, 249
Tylenol: 276
Vaccines: 125, 126
Valium: 274
Visualisation: 31, 100, 106, 151, 318
Vitamin B12: 68, 126, 234, 248
Vitamin C: 23, 54, 121, 249
Walking: 7, 21, 23, 29, 31, 42, 48, 56, 59, 62, 68, 87, 109, 127, 129, 145,
153, 162, 176, 204, 237, 240, 243, 256, 257, 263, 264, 265, 277, 297,
304, 310, 311, 312, 337, 339
Westcare Residential week: 278,
Wheat-free diet: 58, 64, 67, 82, 106, 160, 178, 186, 236, 241, 241, 249,
282, 305, 310
Wheelchair: 4, 6, 7, 8, 15, 16, 26, 28, 39, 46, 60, 62, 82, 87, 153, 208,
213, 216, 217, 233, 239, 240, 276, 277, 278, 279, 343
X-40 Kit: 148,
Yoga: 53, 63, 152, 160, 161, 164, 186, 213, 214, 215, 216, 217, 218, 239,
245, 274, 307, 308, 319, 334, 340

<u>YOUR RECOVERY STORY</u>

When you have a recovery story we would
love to hear from you!

We will be up-dating the Ebook on the website
regularly

<u>www.cfsrecoverystories.com.</u>

and we would like to produce a second issue of this
book.

We would love to include your story

Email: <u>Alex@cfsrecoverystories.com</u>

RECOVERY FROM CFS

50 PERSONAL STORIES

is also available as an E-book

www.cfsrecoverystories.com

Lightning Source UK Ltd.
Milton Keynes UK
11 November 2010

162720UK00002B/2/P